PREFACE

The Fogarty International Center for Advanced Study in the Health Sciences was established as a memorial to the late Congressman John E. Fogarty of Rhode Island. It had been Mr. Fogarty's desire to create within the National Institutes of Health a center for research in biology and medicine dedicated to international cooperation and collaboration in the interest of the health of mankind.

As an institution for advanced study, the Fogarty International Center has embraced the major themes of biomedical research medical education, environmental health, societal factors influencing health and disease, geographic health problems, international health research and education, and preventive medicine. The Center has published proceedings of conferences and seminars devoted to these subjects.

The Fogarty Center endorses the objectives of this interdisciplinary, self-instructional syllabus and is pleased to have provided support for its development.

>   Milo D. Leavitt, Jr., M.D.
>   Director
>   Fogarty International Center
>   National Institutes of Health

v

EDITORS

WENDY H. WADDELL (AAMC Staff, Division of Educational
Resources and Programs)

Ms. Waddell previously administered the AAMC international
student fellowship program (1972-1974) and developed
country-specific materials for the fellows to use prior
to going overseas.

ROBERT G. PIERLEONI, Ed.D. (University of Kansas Office of
Health Sciences Education)

Dr. Pierleoni provides academic consulting to faculty
on the development of instructional materials, the
measurement and evaluation of student progress and the
assessment of teaching effectiveness. He also designs
and conducts faculty development programs and educational
research studies.

EMANUEL SUTER, M.D. (AAMC Staff, Director, Division of
Educational Resources and Programs)

Dr. Suter directed the AAMC Division of International
Medical Education during the development of the course
and has carried overall responsibility for its coordina-
tion, development, testing and revision.

1980

3

ECOLOGIC DETERMINANTS
OF HEALTH PROBLEMS

AUTHORS

MICHAEL M. STEWART, M.D., M.P.H. (Columbia University
College of Physicians and Surgeons and the Columbia
University Center for Community Health Systems)

An internist with particular interest in tropical medicine,
Dr. Stewart has had a rather eclectic international career
including Slavic studies at Oxford, administrative and
medical teaching responsibilities in Thailand, and
responsibility for directing an ambulatory care program
at a busy public hospital in New York City.

RICHARD H. MORROW, JR, M.D. (Harvard School of Public Health)
Currently in Ghana on a two-year assignment, Dr. Morrow
has contributed to the course through his particular
interest in tropical medicine and the ecology of
infectious and parasitic diseases.

THOMAS A. REILLY, M.D. (Mount Sinai School of Medicine
and City Hospital Center at Elmhurst)

An internist with a hospital appointment in the Department
of Ambulatory Care and Community Medicine, City Hospital
Center at Elmhurst, Dr. Reilly also conducts an active
health services research program.

ALLAN G. ROSENFIELD, M.D., F.A.C.O.G. (Columbia University
Center for Population and Family Health)

Drawing on five years of experience in Thailand, Dr.
Rosenfield has contributed substantially to course units
dealing with the relationship between population growth
and health problems.

ROBERT M. SUSKIND, M.D. (Massachusetts Institute of Technology, Clinical Research Center)

Dr. Suskind combines specialty training in pediatrics
and nutrition with international experience in Cameroons,
Senegal and Thailand. He is particularly interested in
the relationship between nutrition and infection and has
contributed to the course in those areas.

ASSOCIATION OF AMERICAN MEDICAL COLLEGES

INTERNATIONAL HEALTH PERSPECTIVES:
An Introduction in Five Volumes

Wendy H. Waddell, Robert G. Pierleoni and Emanuel Suter, Editors

A SELF-INSTRUCTIONAL COURSE

3

ECOLOGIC DETERMINANTS OF HEALTH PROBLEMS

Michael M. Stewart, M.D., M.P.H.

Thomas A. Reilly, M.D.

Richard H. Morrow, Jr., M.D.

Allan G. Rosenfield, M.D., F.A.C.O.G.

Robert M. Suskind, M.D.

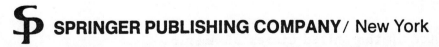 **SPRINGER PUBLISHING COMPANY**/ New York

Development of this international health course was made
possible through the support of the Fogarty International
Center. The information contained in this publication in no
way reflects the views of the Fogarty International Center,
The National Institutes of Health, The Department of Health,
Education and Welfare, or any other Federal agency.

Springer Publishing Company, Inc.
200 Park Avenue South
New York, New York 10003

Library of Congress Catalog Card Number: 77-85140

International Standard Book Numbers: 0-8261-2493-3 (volume 3)
0-8261-2490-9 (5-volume set)

Printed in the United States of America

FOREWORD

For nearly a century, progress in medicine and medical care
has been spearheaded by scientific advances in the biomedical
sciences. The beginning of this era is arbitrarily recognized
with the discoveries of Koch, Pasteur and others--first in
infectious diseases and physiology, and later, in biochemistry.
The culmination of these advances has been the elucidation of
the helical structure for DNA and the recognition of a univer-
sality among elemental biological mechanisms.

Today, major new thrusts in health care are coming from sociocultural, economic and political forces. Every country,
whether old or new, developed or developing, rich or poor,
is confronting problems surrounding the provision of medical
sciences to its people. Serious difficulties are being met
in making health care a right for all people and not a pro-
mise. Escalation of medical care costs around the world
draws more heavily on every nation's resources. The aging
of the world population places a heavier burden on the relatively fewer people in their productive years to meet the
costs of medical care for the aged.

There appears to be no powerful new calculus waiting to be
applied to solve these problems. The equations of the health
economists will not provide answers to essentially moral
questions that center around the difficult issue of how much
of our wealth we will or can spend to relieve human suffering
and preserve human life.

The commonality of the problems makes it essential that all
nations work together in seeking solutions. No country has
an unquestioned preeminence in the field; ideas and solutions
may come from any quarter.

Rapid changes in the health care dynamics of this country and abroad make it desirable for students of medicine to be introduced to issues of health and health care on a worldwide basis. For this reason, the Association has worked with international health faculty throughout the U.S. in producing a course that places U.S. health care against a cross-cultural backdrop of health systems and economic priorities around the world.

The authors and producers of this self-instructional course have employed an ecologic approach to health and disease issues which should help to prepare students both for experience abroad and for health service at home. We in the AAMC are hopeful that these self-instructional materials will prove themselves to be a helpful addition to the educational tools presently available in understanding the health problems that confront us in the United States.

June 1977

JOHN A. D. COOPER, M.D.
PRESIDENT
ASSOCIATION OF AMERICAN
MEDICAL COLLEGES

TABLE OF CONTENTS

The international health course consists of five volumes, each containing independent but related units of content. Throughout the course, the terms "category/volume" are used interchangeably, as are the terms "unit/chapter."

INTRODUCTION

The international health course is expected to serve two functions:

(1) To provide introductory materials for students planning to observe or participate in the health care system of another country, or intending to pursue a career in international health, and

(2) To provide supporting material for some of the community health courses which are being planned or have already been implemented by a number of institutions. (The second title of the course, "Principles of a Cross-Cultural and Comparative Approach to Health Problems," implies that many of the "principles" are presented in an international context, but are equally pertinent to the immediate health concerns of the United States.

The course is designed to stimulate self-learning and to encourage periodic reflection on health problems and concepts through interspersed questioning. Because this self-instructional format makes tutorial guidance by an instructor particularly effective, the course can be used either as a freestanding exercise or in conjunction with other course materials. For faculty who wish to use the course formally within the curriculum, an evaluation packet can be obtained by writing to the Division of Educational Resources and Programs, Association of American Medical Colleges, One Dupont Circle, N.W., Suite 200, Washington, D. C. 20036.

The need for an international health course gradually became apparent to AAMC over a several year period during which the Association sponsored international fellowships for third and fourth year U.S. medical students in other countries. Often, it was learned, U.S. students had difficulty in comparing health information from other countries with our U.S. situation. Repeatedly, these students pointed to the need for better preparation prior to overseas travel.

Following indepth discussions by the Midwest Universities Consortium on International Activities as to the scope and content of such a course, and after more comprehensive discussions with international health faculty at the AAMC Annual Meetings of 1972 and 1973, support for the development of the course was obtained from the Fogarty International Center, National Institutes of Health in May 1975. The course underwent a pilot test phase in early 1977 during which more than 140 students from 15 medical and public health schools used the materials and generated suggestions for this revised first edition.

The development of this international health course was made possible through the efforts of many people over a two year period. In addition to the contributions of our international health experts, we want to thank Dr. Donald Pitcairn of the Fogarty International Center for his continuing support and encouragement. We are grateful to the faculty members and students at fifteen institutions around the country, who agreed to take the course and provide us with constructive criticism for its revision. Dr. James DeNio and Ms. Carol Payne of the University of Kansas Medical Center helped us with the evaluation materials and Ms. Mary Staples of the AAMC provided able and cooperative assistance with all of the administrative details of the project. We also must acknowledge the patience and perseverance of Ms. Veda Tripp in typing the manuscript and Ms. Lesley Knox in tabulating the pilot test results and producing the final typed copy for the these volumes.

WENDY H. WADDELL
Association of American Medical Colleges

ROBERT G. PIERLEONI, Ed.D.
University of Kansas Medical Center

June 1977

EMANUEL SUTER, M.D.
Association of American Medical Colleges

INTRODUCTION TO CATEGORY III

The nine instructional units in Category III, "Ecological Determinants of Health Problems," are intended to serve as a selective introduction to certain of the world's major health problems: diseases of modernization, and urbanization (III/2), infectious and parasitic diseases (III/3 - III/6), population growth (III/7 and III/8) and nutritional disorders (III/9). The total content of these units is by no means comprehensive, and many diseases which are of major importance on a global scale are not discussed (for example, mental illness, cancer and most degenerative diseases). This is partly due to practical limits of time and space, as well as to the particular interests and backgrounds of the authors involved. (It should be noted that the authors of these units have recently spent a combined total of more than 20 years living and working in Thailand and in sub-Saharan Africa, which accounts in part for the frequent references to these settings). Intentional emphasis has been placed on health problems of developing countries, on the assumption that students using this course are likely to be interested in, but relatively unfamiliar with, such areas. These units do not have to be read in strict sequential order, except for III/4-III/5 and III/7-III/8 where an understanding of the material presented in the second unit of the pair requires familiarity with the prior unit.

UNIT III/1. GENERAL ECOLOGICAL CONSIDERATIONS

BY
MICHAEL M. STEWART, M.D., M.P.H.

INTRODUCTION

The range of problems which are appropriate concerns for a student of international health is challenging, even staggering, in scope and complexity. One basic skill which every student of international health should try to cultivate is the ability to construct and continually refine a set of conceptual models that will help to put many different types of information into a perspective which can be used to identify, analyze, and compare different types of health problems in a variety of settings. This first unit in Category III should help you to think in broad conceptual terms about the ecological determinants of certain international health problems.

EDUCATIONAL OBJECTIVES

At the completion of this unit, you will be able to:

1) Draw a schematic diagram indicating two major ecological determinants in the occurrence of malaria, malnutrition, and accidental trauma.

2) Identify, from a list given, those health problems for which the major determinants are those associated with an ecological transition, an ecological disruption, or an ecological niche.

GENERAL ECOLOGICAL CONSIDERATIONS

For purposes of Category III, the following working definition is important:

> medical ecology is the study of humans as members of communities and population groups, in terms of 1) their interactions with their surrounding physical environment (both natural and man-made) and with other living beings (humans and others), and 2) the contributions of these interactions to specific changes in human health status and to the occurrence of particular diseases.

If you have already studied epidemiology, you will note a certain similarity between this definition of medical ecology and one of the standard definitions of epidemiology, which is often said to be the "study of the distribution and determinants of disease in human population groups." The techniques of epidemiology are clearly of central importance for medical ecology, as defined above. We will not be using ecological terms such as "biosphere" and "technosphere" in these units, and no attempt is made to examine or discuss highly technical ecological issues such as net transformation of energy across species boundaries or the impact of human populations on the flora and fauna of the particular ecosystems in which they live. You are not being asked to become an expert in ecology, but rather to think in general ecological terms about the occurrence of important human health problems. You may then wonder, what are the important differences between our working definition of medical ecology and some of the common definitions of epidemiology? Two are suggested. First and most important is the concept that every community health problem has an identifiable ecological setting. Second is the concept that the ecological settings of different types of community health problems can be usefully grouped for comparative analysis.

Appreciation of the first concept ("every community health problem has an identifiable ecological setting") should provide a stimulus for evaluating available epidemiological data on the occurrence of human disease in terms of all the other information you may have about potentially relevant interactions between specific human population groups and their physical, biological and societal* environments.

This is usually an empirical, descriptive and deductive activity, in which classical descriptive epidemiology

---

*Please note another working definition: for purposes of Category III, "societal" means the sum of "social, cultural, political and economic."

plays a necessary but not always sufficient role. The second concept ("ecological settings of community health problems can be usefully grouped and compared") should serve as a challenge for you to try to generalize, to be inductive, and to search for common elements in observed patterns of the occurrence of human diseases and health problems which may be related to important similarities in various ecological settings which initially appear diverse and unrelated. In general, when the phrase "ecological determinants of health problems" is used in these units, it can be interpreted as shorthand for "those physical, biological, and societal factors which influence the occurrence of particular health problems in particular population groups in particular settings during specified time periods."

ECOLOGICAL TRANSITION

Most community health problems in most societies are continuously undergoing gradual changes in incidence, prevalence, community impact and the inter-relationships of different contributing factors. Many (perhaps most) human health problems could therefore be described in terms of gradual ecological transition. This would apply, for example, to many of the factors held responsible for long-term (secular) trends in the frequency of lung cancer among adult males in Europe and North America, or to many of the factors related to the occurrence of health problems already mentioned in Units I/2 and I/3 (for example, see the diagram and related discussion of predominant causes of infant mortality in the U.S. during the period 1900-1930, Unit I/3, p. 13).

It is also important to recognize two more extreme situations which can be important in a comparative approach to international health: the existence of ecological niches and the occurrence of periodic ecological disruptions.

ECOLOGICAL NICHES

Briefly stated, an ecological niche can be defined for our
purposes as a focal, circumscribed geographic setting where
the occurrence of human disease is related to the specific
type and extent of human exposure to a particular set of
physical, biological and/or societal factors which are known
to be determinants of disease. One example would be iodine-
deficiency goiter which is found in particular parts of the
world ("goiter belts") where dietary iodine intake (in food
and water) is unusually low and where supplemental iodine
(such as iodized salt) is not generally used. Other examples
would be the adverse physiological effects of weightlessness
or reduced gravity experienced by astronauts during space
missions and on the surface of the moon, or the occurrence of
scurvy among seamen eating diets deficient in Vitamin C
before the discovery that citrus fruits and juices contained
an important nutrient. Among infectious diseases,
bartonellosis (a bacterial disease transmitted from human to
human by sandflies) is generally limited in its occurrence
to persons living at altitudes between 2,000 and 9,000 feet
in certain countries of South America, since this is the
ecological setting in which sandflies prosper. As another
example, scrub typhus (a rickettsial disease) occurs
primarily among rodents in Southeast Asia where mites are
present to act as an essential biological vector. The entry
of humans (soldiers, farmers, anthropologists and others)
into an ecological niche where scrub typhus naturally occurs
among animals can lead to the occurrence of this disease in
humans, as it frequently did in the U.S. armed forces during
the Vietnam war.

For all of these examples, the pertinent "ecological niche"
can be fairly clearly defined in time and space, and the
risk of human disease is primarily a function of being
present and subject to an identifiable set of ecological
determinants of disease.

ECOLOGICAL DISRUPTIONS

By contrast, major <u>ecological disruptions</u> which directly or indirectly lead to a wide variety of health problems would include sudden natural catastrophes, such as earthquakes, famines, and floods, as well as manmade disasters such as war, major political upheaval, or any form of rapid, unplanned or unexpected physical, biological or societal disruption. Some examples would be the recent severe famine in the Sahel region in West Central Africa, the Guatemala earthquake of 1976, or the mass migration of Moslems out of India after partition in the 1940's. It is worth noting that 1976 was a particularly bad year for earthquakes (China, U.S.S.R., New Guinea, Turkey, Guatemala) and over 35,000 persons are estimated to have died as a direct result. An ecological disruption that occurred on a more limited scale was the Bolivian hemorrhagic fever resulting from DDT-sprayed houses for malaria control resulting in cats dying off due to DDT poisoning. The feline deaths resulted in a marked increase in the rodent population who began to enter human habitations. Mites on the rodents transmitted the etiologic agent to susceptible humans.

These three concepts - ecological transition, ecological disruption, and ecological niche - are suggested as conceptual aids only, to be used in helping you to organize your thinking about many types of health problems in many different places. If you can improve on these conceptual aids or can add to them, you should feel free to do so. It is likely that the more familiar you become with specific international health problems, the more you will recognize the limitations of these concepts and will have to develop your own, more sophiscated approaches.

CHANGING PATTERNS OF DISEASE

To help you collect your thoughts, present knowledge and past experiences about health problems and factors that contribute to their occurrence, the following exercise is offered. It is expected that you may be unable to respond to all of it in detail, but it is important for you to think of these problems in this way. Suggested responses with generous commentary follow.

The following societal factors (among others) have frequently been cited as important influences on the reported occurrence of specific diseases in different countries:

    1) rapid intercontinental air travel
    2) relatively unregulated industrial pollution
    3) rural-to-urban migration patterns
    4) increasing mechanization of agriculture
    5) physical crowding in urban areas
    6) disruption of the traditional family unit
    7) promotion of affluent life styles
    8) large-scale hydroelectric and irrigation
       programs

For each health problem listed below (A-H), write in the blank space the number of at least one factor in the list given above (1-8) which you think may be directly related to an observed increase in the frequency of that health problem in an African, Asian or Latin American country:

    A) schistosomiasis   _____
    B) cholera   _____
    C) obesity   _____
    D) mercury poisoning   _____
    E) tuberculosis   _____
    F) malaria   _____
    G) infant malnutrition   _____
    H) trauma   _____

You are not expected to be familiar with the details of all the material presented in these suggested responses. Many times in this category you may encounter questions that appear to exceed your levels of knowledge about specific details. Try to think in terms of general principles, conceptual models and a comparative approach.

A) schistosomiasis __8__

> Hydroelectric schemes and dam development in places such as Africa have rapidly extended the range of ecological settings conducive to the proliferation of snails (which are essential intermediate hosts in the schistosome life-cycle) and to increasing human contact with water containing the cercarial forms of the schistosomes which are infective for humans (See Unit III/4).

B) cholera __1__

> The Haj, or annual Moslem pilgrimage to Mecca (in Saudi Arabia), brings Moslems from all over the world, many by airplane. It has frequently produced focal epidemics of cholera in temporary living quarters in or near Mecca when human waste disposal and water supplies are inadequate, and infected visitors who are asymptomatic excretors of cholera vibrios (bacteria) in their feces are able to spread the infection to other persons with direct exposure. Other examples of disease occurrence being affected by air travel would be imported cases of malaria and African trypanosomiasis which occur in the United States, after acquisition of infection during foreign travel.

C) *obesity* ___7___

As is well-known, affluence (measured in monetary terms)
may be associated with increased ingestion of calories
and decreased energy expenditure. Obesity is usually
an uncommon problem in developing countries (the reasons
are economic, social, and cultural, as well as physiologic).
However, particularly in urban areas of developing countries, obesity may occur for the same reasons that it
does in the U.S. Obesity in developing countries is not
a major community health problem, but it does exist.

D) *mercury poisoning* ___2___

A recent severe outbreak of community-wide organic
mercury poisoning, directly related to extensive pollution
of community water supplies and food sources in Japan,
is discussed in Unit III/2. There are numerous other
recent examples in the United States of focal occurrence
of health problems related to industrial pollution
(kepone , PBB, ketamide).

E) *tuberculosis* ___5___

Human tuberculosis, caused by <u>Mycobacterium tuberculosis,</u>
occurs with greater frequency under conditions of urban
poverty and crowded home conditions. For example, age-
specific prevalence rates of tuberculin positivity (indicating persons infected by <u>M. tuberculosis,</u> regardless
of the occurrence of clinical signs or symptoms) is often
greater in urban areas of developing countries than in
rural or sparsely-populated areas. Similar patterns
have been observed in urban slums in the U.S. Tuberculosis
is not given major attention in Category III, and you
may wish to pursue this subject with your instructor or
on your own since tuberculosis, while comparatively uncommon in the U.S., is still a major community health
problem in many countries.

F) malaria _1, 4, 8*_

Malaria, a parasitic disease caused by infection with one of four different species of plasmodial protozoans, is more fully discussed in Unit III/6 ("Vector-Borne Diseases"). Here, only the following need be noted:

-malaria may occur as an imported disease, acquired in a distant place but becoming clinically evident in the home country because total time for air travel is shorter than the incubation period for the development of clinical disease.

-increasing mechanization of agriculture and decreasing dependence on domestic beasts of burden may influence mosquito vectors which usually feed on animals to feed more frequently on humans.

-dams and hydroelectric schemes may increase the available sites for multiplication of anopheles mosquito vectors, which breed in water.

G) infant malnutrition _3, 6, 7_

This is discussed in Unit III/9. For now, please note the following points:

-rural-to-urban migration is often accompanied by the need for young mothers to work for cash benefits, and thereby to abandon their responsibilities for breast-feeding and generally nurturing young children during the working day.

*Preferred Response

-disruption of the traditional family unit in any
setting may increase the risk to children,
particularly in terms of priorities in food
distribution and consumption (and also in food and
water hygiene).

-promotion of affluent life styles may influence
parents of infants to substitute bottle-feedings
for breast milk, and to use highly-processed foods
or commercial products (refined sugar, carbonated
beverages) rather than more wholesome natural foods
(breast milk, vegetables, fish) which may be
available at less cost.

H)   trauma ___4___

Trauma and accidents are major causes of death in
many countries among young adults (see Unit III/2).
Injuries may be mechanical (road accidents, use of
new types of heavy equipment), thermal (burns,
usually due to gasoline/kerosene), toxic (due to
careless use of insecticides, rodenticides, etc.),
or the direct result of personal aggression and violence.

UNDERLYING CONCEPT

The frequency of health problems is often related to societal
factors and to specific types of human activity that accompany
technological progress and national socioeconomic development. This general problem of "societal causation of
disease" is by no means limited to highly industrialized
western societies. It exists to some degree in nearly
every country.

You are now asked to consider some physical and biological determinants of human health problems, in contrast to the list of "societal factors" which you have just reviewed. In a general ecological sense, most human activities are affected to some degree by climate, terrain, land use, interactions with other animal species, type and availability of food and water supplies, and man-made environmental incursions. The distribution of health problems is often related to particular elements in the physical and biological environment. These aspects of infectious and parasitic diseases, for example, are discussed in considerable detail in Units III/3 through III/6. In the present unit, the important concept is that all human health problems warrant careful scrutiny in terms of the total ecological context in which they occur, particularly when major determinants of human disease (or "predisposing" and "precipitating causes") can be readily identified in the surrounding environment.

For which of the following diseases (1-6) do you think that annual rainfall and/or prevailing temperature may be an important determinant?   (Write yes or no in the blanks.)

DISEASE	RAINFALL	TEMPERATURE
1) ischemic heart disease	_____	_____
2) hookworm	_____	_____
3) protein-calorie malnutrition	_____	_____
4) malaria	_____	_____
5) lead-poisoning	_____	_____
6) rabies	_____	_____

DISEASE	*RAINFALL*	*TEMPERATURE*
1) *ischemic heart disease*	*no*	*yes*

Exposure to cold temperature can increase metabolic needs and may cause intense vasoconstriction. It is well known that exposure to cold and wind can precipitate attacks of angina pectoris. The clinical advice to a patient with known coronary artery disease to avoid shovelling snow is based on a recognition of combined risks of unusual effort and cold. Although temperature is not recognized as a contributing factor in the pathogenesis of coronary disease, it is clearly involved in its clinical expression.

2) *hookworm*	*yes*	*yes*

Hookworms are parasites passed from human to human. Following excretion of hookworm eggs in feces, hookworm larvae capable of penetrating human skin develop in soil under proper conditions of warmth, moisture and shade. Extremes of dryness, flooding or cold will interrupt this transmission cycle.

3) *protein-calorie malnutrition*	*yes*	*yes*

At the most simplistic level, rainfall in many areas of the world determines the length of the growing and fishing seasons, and therefore directly influences the available family and community food supply. Also, colder temperatures require expenditure of more calories.

DISEASE	RAINFALL	TEMPERATURE
4) *malaria*	*yes*	*yes*

*Each anopheles mosquito vector of malaria has a parti-
cular temperature range within which it is maximally
prolific and effective as a vector. Since mosquitoes
breed in water, rainfall can be an important determinant
of mosquito breeding sites and locations.*

| 5) *lead-poisoning* | *no* | *no* |

*Major sources of human lead exposure are household paint,
vehicle exhausts, and specific industrial exposure. None
of these are critically dependent upon rainfall or temperature although human exposure to a variety of air pollutants
may vary considerably with climatic conditions.*

| 6) *rabies* | *no* | *no* |

*Rabies virus is usually transmitted to man as a result of
the bite of an infected domestic or wild animal with
virus in its saliva. It can occur in nearly any geographic
or climatic setting. Rainfall and temperature are not
directly involved.*

UNDERLYING CONCEPTS

*Physical and biological determinants of human health
may operate independently or in concert. For infections and
parasitic diseases, it is important to consider how the physical environment and climate may affect all elements involved
in the cycle of disease transmission to humans. It is also
important to note that physical and biological determinants
can interact with some of the societal determinants mentioned
previously.*

A GENERAL MODEL FOR OUTLINING HEALTH PROBLEMS

Having considered (even if in a rather superficial way) some
of the wide range of ecological determinants of human health
problems, now review Figure 1 on the next page, which is a
schematic model of the occurrence of human health problems.
As the diagram shows, needs and demands for <u>health care</u> (before disease) and for <u>medical care</u> (after the onset of disease)
can be schematically outlined (steps 1, 1A, 2, 2A, 3, 4, 4A, 5).
Similarly, the general response of the "health care system"
can be outlined in terms of the influence of and interactions
between health sector goals and priorities, policies and specific components of the delivery systems in responding to
community health needs and demands (steps I, II, III and IV).
This diagram is clearly only a rough outline, and for every
community or disease entity which you might want to examine
in detail, this diagram will have to be revised and sharpened.
As a general conceptual model, however, it should prove useful
in helping you to focus on questions such as the following:

1) What is the relative importance of societal vs.
   physical and biologic determinants of health hazards
   and risk factors for specific diseases in different
   communities. For example, is the occurrence of typhoid
   in New York City determined by factors similar to, or
   different from, those factors which are involved in the
   occurrence of typhoid in Mexico or Cairo? If different,
   at what point on the diagram are important determinants
   taking effect?

2) To what degree do specific patterns of health and medical care behavior determine the community impact or
   effectiveness of a national health and medical care
   system for particular communities? For example, does the
   use of intramuscular injections have a particular sociocultural meaning that must be considered in planning vaccination programs? Is this likely to be an important
   societal determinant of disease?

FIGURE 1

SCHEMATIC MODEL OF A HEALTH AND MEDICAL CARE SYSTEM

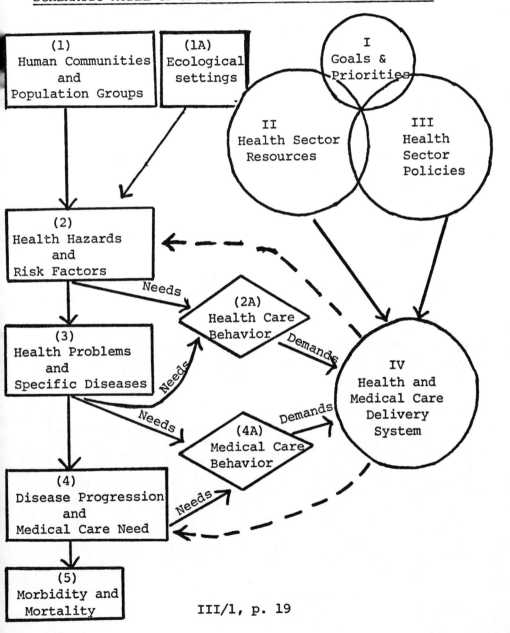

III/1, p. 19

3) How do country-specific health and medical care delivery systems differ in their preventive orientation, as measured by their capacity to identify and respond to the occurrence of health hazards and risk factors (primary prevention), presymptomatic disease (secondary prevention), and clinical illness (tertiary prevention)? Do these differences tend to be disease-specific or more related to the type of national health/medical care delivery system?

4) In settings where specific types of ecological determinants are at work (such as a high prevalence of vector-borne or fecally-transmitted diseases, or in cases where specific causes of trauma or toxic diseases can be identified), do national health sector policies and resources seem to have been deployed in a rational and cost-effective manner?

UNDERLYING CONCEPTS

1) The ecological determinants of health problems can be usefully grouped into physical, biological and societal factors.

2) The occurrence of health problems in different temporal and geographic settings can be usefully compared in terms of the influence of different ecological determinants and the responsiveness of the existing health and medical care system.

For each of the diseases (A, B, C) listed below, write in the blank space the one or two ecological determinants (1-6) which you think may be the MOST important influence on disease occurrence in a "typical" developing country at the present time:

DISEASE   DETERMINANTS

A) malaria   _____   1) a reservoir of infected
                                    humans

B) childhood protein-
   calorie malnutrition ____   2) total family income

C) trauma, accidents   _____ 3) type(s) of local industry

                                4) climate/rainfall

                                5) abundance of vector(s)

                                6) types of farm equipment used

SUGGESTED RESPONSES:

These are the preferred responses, although other determinants listed on page 21 may also apply.

DISEASE	DETERMINANTS
A) malaria	1, 5

Malaria, transmitted from human to human via the anopheles mosquito vector, also requires a substantial reservoir of infected humans for effective transmission to continue.

B) malnutrition	2, 4

Poverty and infant and childhood malnutrition often occur together. As already mentioned, rainfall and climate are related to growing seasons and total food production.

C) trauma, accidents	3, 6

Farm accidents and industrial pollution/toxicity have been mentioned above.

Based on your current knowledge, for each of the diseases/
health problems listed below (A-F), indicate in the blank
space whether you think this is primarily a health problem
of 1) an ecological transition, 2) an ecological disruption,
or 3) an ecological niche.

HEALTH PROBLEMS   TRANSITION/DISRUPTION/NICHE

A) rabies   _____

B) obesity   _____

C) lung cancer   _____

D) severe burns   _____

E) Vitamin C deficiency   _____

F) radiation sickness   _____

SUGGESTED RESPONSES:

These are the preferred responses although others offered on page 23 may also apply.

A) rabies   _ecological niche (3)_

B) obesity   _ecological transition (1)_

C) lung cancer   _ecological transition (1)_

D) severe burns   _ecological disruption (2)_

E) Vitamin C deficiency   _ecological niche (3)_

F) radiation sickness   _ecological disruption (2)_

FINAL NOTE

This introductory unit to Category III is one which you may wish to re-read later as you continue to work on the subsequent units in this Category. Although no list of suggested readings is provided, you may wish to develop your own reference list and your own list of important questions as you progress through Category III and the remainder of the course.

UNIT III/2. HEALTH PROBLEMS OF MODERNIZATION AND URBANIZATION

BY

MICHAEL M. STEWART, M.D., M.P.H.
THOMAS A. REILLY, M.D.

CONTENTS

INTRODUCTION

There are many obvious and important differences between developed and developing countries in terms of disease-specific morbidity and mortality rates. The types of health problems which are given most emphasis in Category III (infectious and parasitic diseases, rapid population growth, and nutritional disorders) are critical community health problems in less developed areas. By contrast, in countries at more advanced stages of socioeconomic development, the leading causes of death usually include cardiovascular diseases, malignancies and various degenerative diseases. Trauma and accidents are notable as leading causes of disability and death in both types of settings.

This unit discusses certain problems of modernization and urbanization which are found both in developed and developing countries. Particular attention is given to environmental contamination and pollution and to the worldwide problem of accidents and trauma. The general goal of this instructional unit is to provide you with specific illustrations of one of the important concepts discussed in Unit III/1: the ecological settings of different types of community health problems can be usefully grouped for comparative analysis.

EDUCATIONAL OBJECTIVES

At the completion of this unit, you will be able to:

1) classify health problems of modernization and urbanization into one of four types: health problems of the <u>community at large</u> or of one or more <u>specific high-risk groups</u>, in relation to either a <u>focal</u> or a <u>diffuse</u> set of ecological determinants.

2) compare the community impact of accidents and trauma as health problems for different population groups in developed and developing countries,

3) identify, from a list provided, those preventive measures which are likely to reduce the frequency of lead poisoning and motor-vechicle injuries.

MODERNIZATION AND URBANIZATION: OVERVIEW

The majority of American citizens usually takes for granted the availability of the "basic necessities" of life: adequate and healthful food; suitable housing; a safe and abundant water supply; relatively clean air; an effective solid and liquid waste disposal system; and relatively cheap and convenient transportation and communication. Moreover, most communities in countries such as the U.S. place a high priority on employment and income opportunities, and on the ready availability of educational, cultural and health services for most citizens.

In many developing countries, however, rapid and unplanned growth in urban areas has created huge squatter settlements with shoddy or makeshift dwellings, often without clean water supplies, without proper toilets, drainage or sewage systems, with inadequate provisions for refuse disposal, without proper roads or even safe foot-paths, and without adequate numbers of community schools, recreation areas, or basic health care facilities.

The adverse effects of these poor basic living conditions are often compounded by factors such as severe and widespread poverty, large and crowded families with inadequate living space and little chance to provide proper care and nutrition for infants and young children, and gross environmental pollution from the discharge of untreated sewage into the nearest water supply, from narrow roads choked with motor vehicles spewing out exhaust fumes, and from careless or negligent conditions in unregulated local industries. A fragile social matrix may also foster the occurrence of problems such as tuberculosis and venereal disease, prostitution, illegal abortion, drug and alcohol addiction, and social unrest accompanied by high rates of crime and personal violence.

To students familiar with severely depressed inner-city areas in the U.S., the above list of adverse conditions will have a familiar ring. However, some of the underlying social processes may be very different in different settings; for example, rapid and unplanned rural-to-urban migration in developing countries, as compared to the recent exodus of the white middle class from central city areas in the U.S., with a dramatic shrinkage in the urban tax base and a shift of social priorities and concerns to the suburbs.* Unfortunately, the net impact for large numbers of urban residents in these two different situations can be distressingly similar: crowding, poverty, social and psychological stress, and ill health.

At the same time that urban conditions of poverty, crowding and slums are taking such a heavy toll, different types of health problems have become prominent among the more privileged and affluent upper classes in many societies. These include premature arteriosclerotic heart disease,

---

* For a different interpretation of the "urban crisis" in the U.S., see Banfield, E.C. "A Critical View of the Urban Crisis," pp. 7-14 in reference 9.

obesity and its sequelae, and increasingly frequent malignant and degenerative diseases which have emerged as major community health problems when environmental and social conditions are such that infectious diseases, mal- nutrition and preventable maternal and child health problems have been effectively reduced.

SUMMARY

List below at least four health problems which you think can be appropriately called "health problems of modernization and urbanization" in developing countries:

1) _____

_____

2) _____

_____

3) _____

_____

4)_____

_____

A number of health problems of modernization and urbanization frequently seen in developing countries have already been mentioned (some are also common in developed countries):

1) *environmental contamination and pollution*
2) *malnutrition, particularly among young children*
3) *communicable diseases (TB. VD. and others)*
4) *alcohol and drug abuse*
5) *trauma and accidents (including violent crime)*

You may also have mentioned some of the following:

6) *gastrointestinal infections*
7) *mental and psychological stress*
8) *occupational hazards*
9) *family disruption and social disorganization*
10) *poverty and its direct effects on health status*

There is no single or all-inclusive list of "correct answers" for this question. What must be stressed is that in many urban areas of the world, basic living conditions are so poor that every individual, family and community group is constantly assaulted by a large number of adverse physical and societal factors and by many toxic exposures and prevalent infectious diseases. The assumed "benefits" of modernization and urbanization may be hard to discern amidst the often depressing conditions of abject poverty, social disorganization and ill health which characterize extensive areas in many of the world's growing number of large cities.

ENVIRONMENTAL CONTAMINATION AND POLLUTION

In recent years, newspapers and magazines have reported numerous dramatic incidents of environmental pollution, some of them directly associated with severe clinical diseases (kepone, polyvinylchloride). We are also confronted with grim details about more pervasive and possibly long-term ecological damage due to careless human activity, such as oil spills (as in the 1967 wreck of the oil tanker Torrey Canyon off the coast of Great Britain, or the wreck of the Argo Merchant near Nantucket in 1976, seriously endangering nearby fishing grounds), damage to the earth's ozone layer, possible radiation hazards from nuclear energy plants, and the poisoning of water resources and wildlife habitats.

As a first step in considering the human health impact of environmental contamination and pollution, it will be useful to use the following simple conceptual framework:

1) Source of environmental contamination:

   Focal
   Diffuse

2) Persons affected:

   Community at large
   Specific high-risk sub-group(s)

LEAD POISONING

For example, lead poisoning of young children is still a serious problem in urban areas where the interior surfaces of houses and apartments are coated with lead-based paint. Recent surveys of blood-lead measurements in urban areas of the U.S. indicate that somewhere between 50,000 and 600,000 children are affected, primarily through ingestion of paint chips, plaster and contaminated soil in settings where white lead had previously been used as an interior pigment (recently manufactured paint usually contains titanium dioxide as a pigment, rather than white lead).

This childhood lead poisoning problem can be classified as due to a <u>diffuse environmental source</u> affecting a <u>specific high risk population group</u>:

Source of Contamination

		Focal	Diffuse
Persons Affected	Community at large		
	High risk group(s)		lead poisoning (children)

By contrast, lead poisoning is also associated with inhalation of heavy concentrations of exhaust fumes of vehicles using lead-containing gasoline. Blood-lead levels have been reported to be twice as high in persons living near major freeways as in other urban residents. Levels are also significantly higher among automobile tunnel workers, and in other settings where there is constant exposure to dense traffic fumes. The pollutant effect of lead in vehicular exhausts makes lead poisoning a potential hazard for all urban residents. Thus lead poisoning from this source can be characterized as due to a <u>diffuse environmental source</u> affecting the <u>community at large</u>:

Source of Contamination

		Focal	Diffuse
Persons Affected	Community at large		lead poisoning (exhaust fumes)
	High risk group(s)		lead poisoning (children)

III/2, p. 8

Further, lead poisoning is a special hazard to certain categories of workers (miners, smelters, workers in battery factories, typesetters, etc.) in settings where lead is being processed, and also to persons eating or drinking from poorly glazed earthenware containers where lead or lead chromate used in the glazing process is leached into the liquid contents.

| | | Source of Contamination | |
		Focal	Diffuse
Persons Affected	Community at large		lead poisoning (exhaust fumes)
	High risk group(s)	lead poisoning (workers; earthenware users)	lead poisoning (children)

It should be obvious, based on even the limited information provided on these different types of lead poisoning, that prevention of lead poisoning will require different types of intervention in various settings, since the determinants of lead poisoning in a given situation can be highly variable.

(You may wish to review the clinical, epidemiologic and preventive aspects of lead poisoning in greater detail, either with your instructor or on your own).

MERCURY POISONING

A dramatic example of environmental contamination occurred in Minimata, Japan in the 1950's and 1960's. Minimata, a quiet fishing village located on the southern Japanese island of Kyushu, had for many years been the site of a large chemical factory providing employment to villagers. In the early 1950's a strange "dancing disease" with frequent deaths was noted among village cats, along with unexplained

deaths among pigs, dogs, seabirds, fish and shellfish.
In early 1956, an 11 month-old girl was admitted to the
local factory hospital with a severe, unexplained neurological syndrome (delerium, speech and gait disturbances),
and it was determined that some 30 other children and
adults, including friends and neighbors, were also affected.
This illness, quickly named "Minamata Disease," was at
first thought to be infectious in origin, but by late 1956
a form of heavy metal poisoning was strongly suspected.
Among the agents considered were manganese, thallium,
selenium, arsenic, organic mercury, or a combination of
these toxic metals.

Symptoms in affected humans usually included numbness in
the extremities, difficulty executing fine movements,
weakness, tremors, ataxia, dysarthria, and gradual impairment of sight and hearing. Of the first 52 cases discovered,
21 patients died (20 within six months of clinical
detection).

Attention quickly focused on the chemical plant and the
waste materials which it discharged daily into Minamata
Bay. Despite strong resistance and a continuing lack of
cooperation from factory officials, aggressive investigation gradually proved that inorganic mercury, used as a
catalyst in the production of acetaldehyde and polyvinylchloride, was being methylated in the production process
and then discharged into the bay in large amounts. This
organic form of mercury readily entered the aquatic food
chain, and was subsequently consumed by humans (and animals)
in fish and shellfish, the main local sources of dietary
protein. By the end of 1962 there were 121 officially
verified cases, with 46 deaths.

Indicate on the diagram below (in the spaces 1-4) the type(s) of environmental health problem illustrated by this outbreak of methyl-mercury poisoning:

<u>Source of Contamination</u>

	Focal	Diffuse
Community at large	(1)	(2)
<u>Persons Affected</u> High risk group(s)	(3)	(4)

Source of Contamination

	Focal	Diffuse
Community at large	(1) methyl-mercury poisoning	(2) ?
High risk group(s)	(3) ?	(4) ?

Persons Affected

Based on the information provided, this is primarily (1), a problem of environmental contamination of <u>focal origin</u> affecting the <u>community at large</u>. However, you might also have correctly checked boxes 2 and 3:

(2) Once methyl-mercury found its way into the aquatic food chain (particularly fish), it inevitably became an immediate health hazard for everyone living in a wide geographic area.

(3) Methyl-mercury ingestion was particularly great among persons living closest to the site of sludge discharge from the chemical factory, since fish and shellfish in that immediate area had higher concentrations of mercury, as measured in ppm (parts per million).

One further aspect of this outbreak of methyl-mercury poisoning which was not appreciated for several years was the occurrence of congenital Minamata Disease: relatively asymptomatic pregnant women ingesting contaminated seafood frequently gave birth to children with mental retardation, seizure disorders and severe cerebellar symptoms (between 1955-1958, some 6% of all children born in Minamata were so affected). Methyl-mercury, even at relatively low blood levels, readily passes the placenta and is particularly damaging to the developing fetal nervous system.

One of the most tragic and distressing aspects of this episode of environmental contamination and ensuing human disease was the protracted delay in correcting the basic problem. The chemical factory continued to discharge methyl-mercury into Minamata Bay until 1968, and the final toll in terms of cases of "verified" disease numbered in the hundreds. The story of Minamata Disease represents a classic and instructive conflict between the health interests of a local community and the profit motives (and community employment benefits) of an industrial corporation. This same conflict, now often phrased in terms of "social vs. economic trade-offs," can be identified in many current controversies over attempts to regulate various industrial wastes (see reference #12 for details of Minamata Disease).

ASBESTOS

We now shift briefly to a more subtle and widespread problem of industrial contamination, that of asbestos. Asbestos is the generic name for a variety of naturally-occurring mineral silicates which are widely used in modern industry for purposes that require resistance to heat and friction, tensile strength and flexibility. Some of the major uses of asbestos include insulation and fireproofing, cement, brake linings, talc, air conditioning ducts and special fabrics.

Exposure to asbestos (in its various forms) has been shown to be directly associated with the development, after many years, of at least three types of health problems: fibrotic disease of the lungs (asbestosis), malignant disease of the pleura and peritoneum (mesothelioma), and primary lung cancer. It has recently become evident that "exposure to asbestos" is a complex and pervasive phenomenon. Exposure can occur as an occupational hazard (among pipe-fitters, construction workers, auto mechanics, etc.), among families of workers who inadvertently contaminate their home environments with asbestos fibers from their clothes, and among "asbestos neighbors" or persons living in the immediate vicinity of factories where asbestos is used in a manufacturing process, and may be discharged into the ambient air. There also is evidence that industrial discharge of asbestos-containing wastes into community water supplies may be producing significant and dangerous levels of asbestos in drinking water (current water treatment methods do not specifically eliminate asbestos).

Indicate on the diagram below the type(s) of environmental health problem(s) (1-4) illustrated by these various types of asbestos contamination and pollution:

	Source of Contamination	
	Focal	Diffuse
Persons Affected — Community at large	(1)	(2)
Persons Affected — High risk group(s)	(3)	(4)

Source of Contamination

	Focal	*Diffuse*
Community at large	*(1)* *factory discharge of asbestos into air*	*(2)* *asbestos in drinking water*
High risk group(s)	*(3)* *asbestos in closed environment (factory, home, garage, etc.)*	*(4)*

Persons Affected

(You may wish to pursue the important subject of asbestos pollution in greater detail with your instructor or on your own).

ACCIDENTS AND TRAUMA

OVERVIEW

Accidents and trauma represent a neglected epidemic in the modern world. The United Nations recently estimated that accidents are the third ranking cause of death worldwide, with the automobile playing a major role in accidental deaths. In the United States, 25% of all persons are accidentally injured each year (some 50% of all such injuries require medical treatment). The 1972 U.S. National Health Survey indicated that 11.5 million persons were temporarily disabled due to accidents, 420,000 were permanently disabled, and 117,000 persons died of accidental causes. Accidents in the U.S. in 1972 were the fourth-ranking cause of death overall, accounting for 7.5% of total mortality, and accidents were the leading cause of death in the age group 0-45 years. Similar patterns are observed in many other countries.

Accidents can be conveniently grouped by type of injury into two major groups: those due to the imposition of excess external energy on the human body, and those due to impairment of physiologic energy exchange (see Table 1).

TABLE 1

Type of Injury

1) Energy exceeding local/whole-body threshold
   - mechanical (displacement, breakage, crushing)
   - thermal (inflammation, charring, coagulation)
   - electrical (burning, neuromuscular disturbance)
   - ionizing radiation (disruption of cellular function)

2) Interference with energy exchange
   - oxygen utilization (suffocation, CO poisoning)
   - thermal control (frost-bite, heatstroke)

The great majority of accidents fall into the "excess energy" category. In the U.S. in 1973, there were 117,000 accidental deaths. Of these, 14,100 occurred in the work place, 27,000 in the home, 24,300 in public situations (including recreation), and 51,600 deaths were attributable to motor vehicle accidents (MVA's).

FIGURE 1

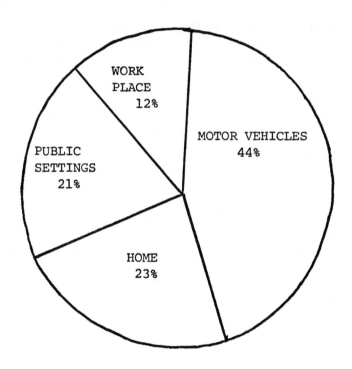

Proportional Accident Mortality by Site of Accident, U.S.
1973

III/2, p. 18

MOTOR VEHICLE ACCIDENTS

Since the invention of motor vehicles at the start of the
20th century, there has been an exponential increase in
MVA mortality figures. Young males (age 15-35) are at
particular risk of death from this cause. For example, in
the U.S. in 1973, 37% of all male deaths in the age group
20-29 were due to motor vehicle accidents (as compared to
19% of female deaths in the same age group, and only 2% of
all male deaths in the age group 50-59). Since 1965,
there have been more than 1.7 million deaths in the U.S.
from vehicular accidents, a total far exceeding the number
of American deaths in any war. Moreover, the loss of
working years due to MVA's (U.S., 1971) represents some
6.5% of the total working years lost from all causes of
death in the U.S., whereas accidents account for only about
3% of all deaths. A more comforting statistic , perhaps,
is that the death rate per number of vehicular miles
travelled has fallen in the U.S. over the past 50 years
from 25.3 per billion to 5.4 per billion.

It is important to realize that MVA's are rapidly becoming
an important health problem in developing countries.
In Taiwan, for example, as socioeconomic conditions have
progressed and the numbers of vehicles and roads have
increased, the MVA death rate is rising as the crude death
rate and death rate from infectious diseases are falling,
so that MVA's are responsible for an increasing proportion
of all deaths (now about 1.2% of all deaths, as compared to
3% in the U.S.).

This rise in MVA death rates in developing countries has many contributing causes: poor road systems, inadequate driver education, ineffective traffic control and vehicle safety codes, and other factors. However, probably the most important factors are the increasingly large number of vehicles on the road and the greater number of miles travelled.

Indeed, it has been suggested that the number of MVA injuries can be roughly predicted by using the following formula:

MVA casualties $\approx 0.0003 \ (V \times P)^{1/3}$

where V = number of vehicles
P = total population

Indicate which of the other factors below (1-5) you think
may be directly related to the accidental death rate in
any given society (answer yes or no):

Factors	Related ?
1) age	_____
2) sex	_____
3) rural vs. urban sites	_____
4) education	_____
5) social class	_____

Possibly-Related Factors	Related (Yes/No)
1) age	_yes_
2) sex	_yes_
3) rural vs. urban sites	_yes_
4) education	_yes_
5) social class	_yes_

Sex and age appear to be the factors most closely related to accidental death rates, at least in developed countries. For MVA's, for example, there is a striking peak in the death rate for males in the age group 20-29, as already noted. Actually, for the male age group 15-24 in the U.S., the figure is even more dramatic: 70% of deaths in this group are due to MVA's. In the U.S. women in the same age group (15-24), MVA's account for only 15% of all deaths.

It is interesting that MVA mortality rates for U.S. males in rural areas are far higher than for males of comparable age groups in urban and suburban areas. Education and socioeconomic class are also associated with MVA mortality rates in the U.S.: mortality rates from MVA's are much higher among poorer and less educated persons, as compared to affluent persons and college graduates (see Table 2).

TABLE 2

DIFFERENTIAL MORTALITY RATIOS*
by Education and Economic Class
(MVA's, U.S.A., 1972)

EDUCATION	MORTALITY RATIO	ECONOMIC CLASS	MORTALITY RATIO
No High School	1.13	I (low)	1.80
Some High School	1.06	II	1.14
High School Grad.	1.01	III	0.81
College Grad.	0.66	IV (high)	0.48

Accidents in the home and in public places accounted for some
44% of all accidental deaths in the U.S. in 1973. Death from
domestic accidents is usually highest at the two extremes of
age. The death rate from domestic accidents in England and
Wales in 1970, for example, was 71/100,000 for persons 65
and over, as compared to 13.3/100,000 for the total population.
"Falls" account for over 40% of deaths in this age group.
Older persons often have poor sight, hearing and balance, and
their diminished mobility can make it difficult to escape
serious personal injury when even a minor accident does occur.

OCCUPATIONAL ACCIDENTS

Occupational accidents are another important category,
accounting for about 12% of all accidental deaths in the U.S.
Reform of labor conditions came late in human history (the
English Factory Act of 1833 was the first effective industrial
legislation). Presently there is concentrated attention on
problems of occupational health and safety in all developing

---

*"Mortality ratio" is the ratio of the mortality rate for
one sub-group as compared to the mortality rate for the
population as a whole. A mortality ratio greater than 1.0
therefore indicates "excess mortality."

countries. However, even today, factory conditions in many developing countries are largely unregulated from a health viewpoint. In developed countries, a concern for occupational health leads to questions such as:

1) to what degree do specific occupations and working environments represent health hazards?

2) do particular occupations exacerbate underlying diseases?

3) how seriously do minor worker illnesses impair work efficiency and increase the hazards of the work environment?

In general terms, occupational hazards can be reduced by three types of efforts: 1) environmental monitoring and epidemiological surveillance; 2) health education of the worker; 3) legislation and regulatory enforcement.

By analogy, these three types of effort might also be usefully applied to other serious community health problems, such as motor vehicle accidents and lead poisoning.

'or each of two problems, lead poisoning and motor vehicle
accidents, identify from the list provided (A-F) the type(s)
of intervention which you feel would specifically help to
reduce the extent of the problem:

Problem	Possible Interventions
1) lead poisoning _____	A) proper highway construction
2) MVA's _____	B) community health education
	C) use of no-lead gasoline
	D) national legislation
	E) 55 mph speed limit
	F) education of high risk groups

1) *lead poisoning* _____ B, C, D, F _____

2) *MVA's* _____ B, D, E, F _____

FINAL NOTE

Obviously the many health problems accompanying urbanization and modernization have been discussed in a highly selective way and have only been sketched in outline. A list of references is provided for further reading in several areas touched on in this unit. Occupational health and safety is a particularly important area which you are urged to explore more fully, particularly since it involves the provisions of medical care to individual patients, as well as a larger concern for epidemiologic surveillance, prevention, and health maintenance. Occupational health on an international scale is a critically important area, and should be of major concern to students.

UNDERLYING CONCEPTS

1. *Modernization and urbanization are global phenomena accompanied by particular types of health hazards.*

2. *Health problems due to environmental contamination and pollution can be initially grouped into those due to <u>focal</u> or <u>diffuse</u> determinants as they affect the <u>community at large</u> or <u>specific high-risk sub-groups.</u>*

3. *Motor vehicle accidents play a major role in the world-wide increase in accidental deaths.*

SUGGESTED FURTHER READING

1. ACPM Task Force, <u>Preventive Medicine USA: Theory Practice and Application of Prevention in Environmental Health Services; Social Determinants of Human Health</u>, PRODIST, New York, 1976.

2. Doxiadis CA: The Inhuman City. Chapter 10 in <u>Health of Mankind</u>, Ciba Foundation Symposium, Little Brown, 1976.

3. Dubos R: Environmental Pollution. Chapter VIII in <u>Man Adapting</u>, Yale University Press, 1965.

4. Eidsvold G et al: The New York City Department of Health: Lessons in a Lead Poisoning Control Program. <u>Amer. J. Public Health</u> 64:956-962, 1974.

5. Ford AB, <u>Urban Health in America</u>, Oxford University Press, 1976.

6. Hobson W, (Editor), <u>The Theory and Practice of Public Health</u> (4th edition), Oxford University Press, 1975 (especially Chapter 28, "Accidents and their Prevention," and Chapter 38, "Occupation and Health").

7. Hughes JP, (Editor), <u>Health Care for Remote Areas</u>, Kaiser Foundation International, 1972 (especially Part Three, "Health Services on Development Projects").

8. Levine RJ et al: Occupational Lead Poisoning, Animal Deaths and Environmental Contamination at a Scrap Smelter. <u>Amer. J. Public Health</u> 66:548-552, 1976.

9. Mott GF, (Special Editor), "Urban Change and the Planning Syndrome," <u>Annals of the American Academy of Political and Social Science</u>, Vol. 405, (January) 1973.

10. Plessas DJ: Environmental Pollution, Social Costs, and Health Policy in the United States. <u>Inter. J. Health Services</u> 4:273-284, 1974.

11. Shy CM: Environmental Pollution in Industrializing Countries. In <u>Community Medicine in Developing Countries</u>, A.R. Omran, Editor, Springer, 1976.

12. Smith WE and Smith AM, <u>Minamata</u>, Holt, Rinehart and Winston, 1975.

13. Waldbott GL, <u>Health Effects of Environmental Pollutants</u>, C.V. Mosby Co., 1973.

14. Ward B and Dubos R, <u>Only One Earth</u>, W.W. Norton Co., New York, 1972 (especially Part Four, "The Developing Regions")

UNIT III/3. BACTERIAL AND VIRAL DISEASES

BY

MICHAEL M. STEWART, M.D., M.P.H.*

CONTENTS

*The author wishes to acknowledge the assistance of
Dr. Richard H. Morrow, Jr.

INTRODUCTION

Environmental factors and patterns of human behavior are major determinants of the frequency and distribution of bacterial and viral diseases in human population groups. These factors can also affect the simultaneous occurrences of different infectious diseases or the reoccurrence of a given infection in the same individual, as well as patterns of naturally-acquired immunity. This instructional unit presents certain basic concepts that will be useful in identifying and comparing the determinants of selected bacterial and viral diseases in different settings. Obviously, given the many hundreds of human bacterial and viral diseases, this unit can focus only on a few illustrations of these concepts as they apply to the epidemiology, community impact, and control of human infections. (Note: This unit is not intended as a substitute for, or review of, a basic course in microbiology. Although such a course is not a prerequisite for this unit, some prior knowledge of microbiology will be very helpful).

EDUCATIONAL OBJECTIVES

At the completion of this unit, you will be able to:

1) Name the elements in a schematic diagram showing the major steps in the transmission of bacterial and viral infections to humans.

2) Use the schematic diagram to group a number of bacterial and viral infections according to their similarities and dissimilarities at different points in the transmission process.

3) Use this schematic diagram to identify those points at which different types of preventive measures take effect.

HOW INFECTIONS ARE ACQUIRED:
SOME GENERAL CONSIDERATIONS

There are only a limited number of ways in which humans can acquire bacterial and viral infections. For example, rubella can result from close personal contact with respiratory aerosols or nasopharyngeal secretions from an infected person, or from transplacental bloodstream infection from mother to fetus. Plague, in its bubonic form, is arthropod-borne, being transmitted by fleas from rodents to man, while pneumonic plague (which is more serious but much less frequent) spreads directly from person to person by inhalation. Typhoid, which only affects humans, is transmitted by what is often called the "fecal-oral route, " usually through ingestion of a food or water source contaminated with human fecal matter. Smallpox, now almost eradicated, spreads only from human to human, primarily by the respiratory route following close personal contact with an acutely infected person or with contaminated fomites (linen, clothes, etc.), although small outbreaks have occurred from virus inhalation at greater distances by persons not in direct contact either with a case of smallpox or with contaminated fomites.

Staphylococcal skin infections in the hospital are often spread by the contaminated hands or the nasal secretions of hospital staff.

This suggests that one useful way to classify bacterial and viral infections is according to the way in which they are acquired by humans, i.e., by inhalation, by ingestion, through skin or mucous membranes, or by transplacental spread.*

---

*Transplacental spread will not be further discussed in this unit.

PREASSESSMENT

For each of the diseases listed at the left below, write in
the blank space the way(s) in which humans commonly acquire
the infection. You will have an opportunity to review your
responses to this exercise before proceeding with the remainder of the unit.

_____1) Diphtheria   A)   inhalation

_____2) Measles   B)   ingestion

_____3) Cholera   C)   skin/mucous membranes

_____4) Poliomyelitis

_____5) Tetanus

_____6) Rabies

_____7) Botulism

_____8) Anthrax

_____9) Tularemia

_____10) Leptospirosis

<u>SUGGESTED RESPONSES</u>:

1) <u>A,C</u>. Diphtheria, a disease which is limited to humans, is acquired from close personal contact, either via respiratory droplets or by direct skin contact. Diphtheria bacilli can produce severe upper respiratory tract infections, and also primary skin ulcers and secondary wound infections. Pathogenic organisms produce a potent exotoxin which causes severe local inflammation, and can also affect cardiac and neural tissues.

2) <u>A,C.</u> Measles virus is acquired by inhalation of infected droplets or by close personal contact with contaminated nasopharyngeal secretions. Systemic infection occurs, usually with skin and respiratory findings predominating. Humans and monkeys are the only known hosts.

3) <u>B.</u> Cholera is acquired by mouth from contaminated food or water. The bacteria (<u>Vibrio cholerae</u>) do not penetrate the intestinal wall, but produce an exotoxin acting on the GI mucosa to cause rapid loss of fluid and electrolytes, often leading to shock or death if untreated. Cholera affects only humans.

4) <u>B.</u> Poliomyelitis is a viral disease spread primarily by the fecal-oral route. Paralytic polio is a relatively infrequent but serious result of human infection. No other animals are involved.

5) <u>C.</u> Tetanus is acquired by direct inoculation into subcutaneous tissues of the spores of <u>Clostridium tetani</u>. Tetanus spores occur naturally in soil, and any skin injury can serve as a point of entry. The bacteria multiply anaerobically, which favors their growth in necrotic tissue. Infection itself is benign, but the bacteria can produce a potent exotoxin with neuro-muscular effects, causing clinical disease.

6) _C._ Rabies is an almost always fatal illness which usually follows the bite of an infected domestic or wild animal
with rabies virus in its salivary secretions. The risk
of human-to-human transmission is close to zero.

7) _B._ Botulism is not really an infectious disease, but
rather is the neurological syndrome caused by ingestion
of the extraordinarily potent botulinum toxin, usually
from food contaminated with the common soil bacterium
Clostridium botulinum. Botulism is the most severe form
of "food-poisoning."

8) _A,C._ Anthrax, caused by _Bacillus anthracis,_ is usually
acquired by direct contact with infected animals or
their hides, or by inhalation of anthrax spores, for
example, in industrial settings where contaminated
animal hides or bones are being processed.

9) _A,B, C._ Tularemia is caused by the bacterium
Francisella tularensis, usually following direct skin
contact with infected animals or their excreta, or
from the bite of an infected arthropod vector. It also
can follow ingestion of contaminated meat or water, or
the inhalation of contaminated aerosols.

10) _C._ Leptospirosis is caused by many different serotypes
of leptospires (bacteria), and usually follows direct
contact of skin or mucous membranes with water contaminated by the urine of an infected animal.

Depending on your prior knowledge of microbiology and virology,
you may have had some difficulty answering the above question,
and you were certainly not expected to know or recall all the
details given with the suggested responses. Now take a moment
to compare your responses on page 5 to the information provided
above on pages 6 and 7. On reading through these suggested
responses, it should be apparent that classifying human infections according to the three categories (A-C) of "how
acquired" is not really an adequate method, since these categories refer only to the routes by which the organism gains

entry into the human body (often termed the "portal of entry").
A more complete picture of the transmission and acquisition of
these ten diseases involves additional considerations such
as the following:

1) some infections have multiple portals of entry
2) some infections are limited to humans
3) animal reservoirs play differing roles
4) some infections are transmitted by arthropod vectors
5) some disease agents occur naturally in soil
6) bacterial toxins play variable roles

In order to put these and other considerations into more clear
perspective, a better conceptual model is needed for outlining
the major steps involved in transmission and acquisition of
human infections.

A SCHEMATIC MODEL

Several sequential steps in the transmission and acquisition
of human infections are illustrated in Figure 1. As indicated
in this schematic model, organisms which infect humans must
physically pass from a reservoir (an infected human or animal,
or in some cases the natural environment) through a portal of
exit into or onto a vehicle of transmission, by which they reach
a portal of entry into the human host. Here the organism may
produce a benign carrier state or it may progress to infection
and disease. Human infection does not necessarily mean disease,
since some persons may have clinically undetectable infections,
and chronic asymptomatic carrier states may follow certain infections. Finally, depending on the infection, a person with
a carrier state, a subclinical infection or a clinical disease
may further transmit the infecting agent via a portal of
exit.

Use of this schematic model makes it simpler to compare and
discuss the various environmental and societal determinants
of a wide variety of human infections. This model is

admittedly a vast oversimplification of many complex biological phenomena, and for certain infections you may have to stretch the conceptual steps in the diagram a bit in order to fit the actual details of transmission. However, it should help you to organize your thinking as a preliminary to later, more detailed study of the epidemiology and ecology of infectious diseases.

FIGURE 1

SCHEMATIC MODEL OF THE TRANSMISSION OF HUMAN INFECTIONS

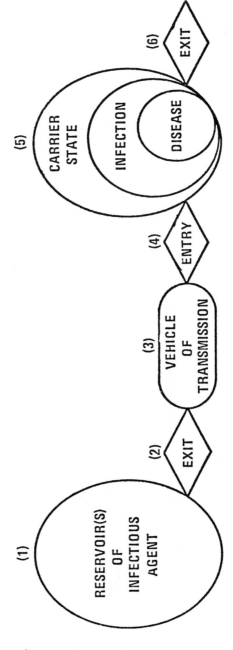

The information already provided for typhoid is diagrammed in Figure 2. This figure summarizes the fact that this infection spreads from human to human via the fecal-oral route through contaminated food or water, and also indicates that both diseased persons and asymptomatic carriers (infected but not diseased) can further transmit typhoid bacteria.

FIGURE 2

TRANSMISSION OF TYPHOID

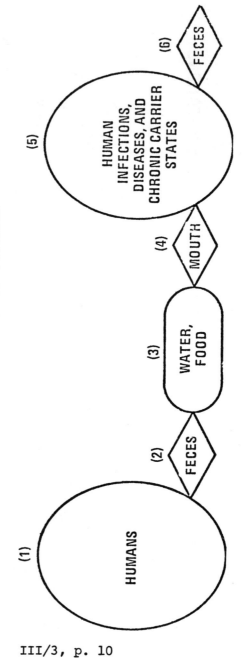

Now try to fill in the blanks for Figure 3 as a schematic model of rabies transmission, using the information provided on pages 6 and 7 (or any other knowledge you may have about rabies).

FIGURE 3

TRANSMISSION OF RABIES

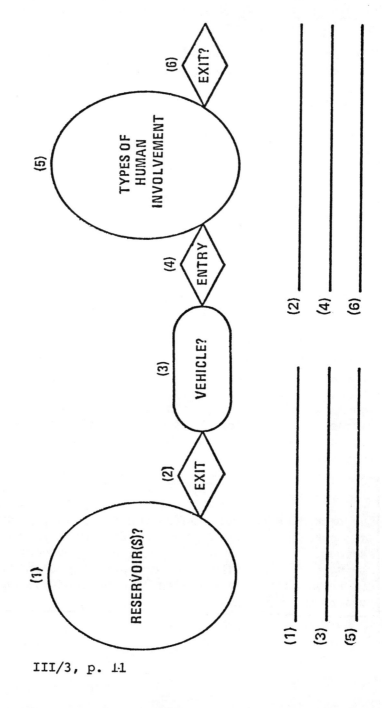

SUGGESTED RESPONSES:

(1) _Reservoirs_ - _infected animals_ of many types, domestic and wild (particularly dogs, bats and skunks).

(2) _Portal of exit_ - _mouth_ of the biting animal

(3) _Vehicle of transmission_ - _saliva of infected animals_

(4) _Portal of entry_ - _human skin_ at the bite site

(5) _Human involvement_ - a lethal non-transmissible infection.

(6) _Portal of exit_ - _none_ (although rabies virus may appear in the saliva of persons with rabies, shedding of virus or infection of another human occurs rarely, if ever)

You may have discovered some of the limitations of this schematic model in answering the question on rabies. For example, the infected animal reservoir might also be considered the vehicle of transmission, bringing the virus directly into contact with a human. Nevertheless, the virus must still exit from the animal, and enter the human in animal saliva. Now, using some scratch paper try to draw schematic models for some of the other infections already discussed. Feel free to make any modifications in this schematic model which are helpful to you (there is no "perfect" diagram).

UNDERLYING CONCEPT

The transmission and acquisition of bacterial and viral pathogens can be schematically diagrammed into a number of sequential steps, providing a general framework for comparing different infections and grouping them according to how these steps are affected by environmental and social factors in different settings.

THE RANGE OF HOSTS FOR PARTICULAR INFECTIONS

Some bacterial and viral agents infect only humans, some infect humans and other animals equally effectively, and some are primarily causes of animal diseases, with humans involved only incidentally (or accidentally). Infections which are commonly present in non-human animal populations are termed enzootic (the comparable term for human infections is endemic). Infections which occur with unusually high frequency among animals are termed epizootic (cf. epidemic for human infections). Animals which are hosts for a given disease agent can also act as reservoirs from which the infection is transmitted to humans. We have already mentioned tularemia, leptospirosis and rabies as examples of bacterial and viral zoonoses (diseases of animals transmitted to man).* For such diseases a full understanding of the occurrence of human infections requires careful consideration of the animal reservoirs involved and of the type and extent of human-animal contact needed for human infection.

Some other zoonoses caused by bacterial or viral agents include:

1) brucellosis (Brucella spp.)

2) salmonellosis (Salmonella spp. other than S. typhosa)

3) equine encephalitis (various arboviruses)

4) plague (Yersinia pestis)

5) relapsing fever (Borrelia spp.)

---

*In a purely technical sense, a "zoonosis" is a disease of animals other than humans. For simplicity's sake, we are using the term in its broader sense, as a natural disease of animals which is also transmitted to humans.

For many zoonoses, human infection occurs primarily through close personal contact with animals or animal excreta (rabies and leptospirosis, for example). Animal excreta may contaminate food supplies (salmonellosis can result from eating contaminated poultry eggs). In other zoonoses, an arthropod vector feeds on infected animals and then on susceptible humans (tularemia, plague). Because the variations in animal habitats and in human-animal contacts are so great, the risk of human infection is critically dependent on local ecological factors and on specific patterns of human behavior. Although this topic will not be discussed further in detail in this unit, you may want to consider: What zoonoses, if any, present significant risks to persons in different areas in the United States? What zoonoses do you think were diagnosed in the past year in the hospitals associated with your medical school? What could have been done to prevent these infections? Are any population groups at particular risk of acquiring zoonotic infections in your own geographic area? Does the existing epidemiologic surveillance system (local, state, national) routinely identify human infections which result from human-animal contact?

Since the topic of zoonoses usually receives only limited attention in medical school curricula, you may wish to pursue these and other related questions on your own.

Now use your current knowledge of microbiology and epidemiology to try to name at least three bacterial and/or viral agents which naturally infect <u>only humans</u> and for which the <u>reservoir</u> in our schematic diagram must therefore always be "humans:"

1)

2)

3)

SUGGESTED RESPONSES:

Organisms for which man is the only natural host and therefore the only reservoir include (among others):

1) _Salmonella typhosa (typhoid)_
2) _Neisseria gonorrheae (gonorrhea)_
3) _Bordetella pertussis (whooping cough)_
4) _Mumps virus (mumps)_
5) _Corynebacterium diphtheriae (diphtheria)_
6) _Smallpox virus (smallpox)_
7) _Vibrio cholerae (cholera)_
8) _Mycobacterium leprae (leprosy)_ *

(If your answer included any agents not listed above, you may wish to consult a microbiology text for confirmation).

The agents listed above, which have no natural host other than man, can be divided into two general groups: those usually communicated during close personal contact with skin or secretions or by respiratory aerosols (gonococci, B. pertussis, mumps virus, diphtheria bacilli, smallpox virus, leprosy bacilli), and those which are usually disseminated without close personal contact, through vehicles of transmission in the environment (typhoid bacilli, cholera vibrios). For both groups, the continuing transmission of infection is greatly facilitated by the existence of carriers, or infected persons who do not have clinical disease but from whom the organisms find a ready portal of exit. Among the diseases listed, leprosy is distinctive in that the clinical infection is a chronic one, and persons with recognized, symptomatic lepromatous leprosy continue to act as sources of contagion to other persons for long periods of time. (They probably are also contagious to other persons well before the disease is clinically recognized). Smallpox is a special case and is further discussed later in the unit.

---

*M. leprae has also recently been shown to occur among armadillos.

SOIL INHABITANTS

Cetain bacteria are common and widespread inhabitants of soil. These include, for example, Clostridium tetani (tetanus), Clostridium botulinum (botulism), Pseudomonas pseudomallei (melioidosis), and Actinomyces israeli (actinomycosis). Some important pathogenic fungi (Coccidioides immitis and Histoplasma capsulatum) are also common soil inhabitants in certain localities and can produce severe human illness when spores are inhaled. However, fungal diseases will not be further discussed in this unit.

Melioidosis is an instructive example of a bacterial infection caused by a common soil inhabitant. The Gram-negative bacterium Pseudomonas pseudomallei is prevalent in Asian soil (South Vietnam, Cambodia, Thailand, India) and has also been found in other parts of the world. Human infection can occur by inhalation, ingestion or through minor skin wounds. Inhalation often causes an acute lower respiratory illness, after which patients may develop chronic cavitary disease of the lungs which mimics tuberculosis. Disseminated melioidosis also occurs, but infrequently. Prior to U.S. involvement in the Vietnam war, American physicians were generally unfamiliar with melioidosis. However, during troop activities in Vietnam, and particularly where helicopters produced severe drafts and soil disturbances, members of the U.S. forces were heavily exposed by inhalation. Many military patients who developed chronic pulmonary disease were thought to have tuberculosis (which is also common in Vietnam), and were returned home to V.A. hospitals, where the true diagnosis was found to be melioidosis. This illustrates the unusual occurrence of a pattern of human disease following entry of a susceptible population group into a circumscribed ecological setting where a particular disease agent was highly prevalent in soil and where one particular portal of entry (the respiratory route) was greatly enhanced by unusual patterns of human behavior.

VECTOR-BORNE DISEASES

Many diseases of humans and other animals are transmitted by arthropods vectors which feed on vertebrate blood.* These include parasitic diseases such as malaria and filariasis, various rickettsioses, and many others. At this point it is important only to note that there are many viruses and a few bacteria which are also vector-borne, for example:

Arboviruses (yellow fever, dengue, equine encephalitis, hemorrhagic fever, etc.)

Francisella tularensis (tularemia)

Borrelia recurrentis (relapsing fever)

Arboviruses are by their very definition dependent on vectors for continuing transmission (ARBOVIRUS = ARthropod-BOrne VIRUS). More than 50 arboviruses are currently known to be pathogenic for man, and most arboviruses have well-defined animal reservoirs, some of them very extensive geographically.

---

*In this unit, arthropod vectors are conceptually regarded as one of the "vehicles of transmission." A more careful distinction between mechanical and biological vectors is made in Unit III/6, "Vector-Borne Diseases."

Tularemia, caused by the Gram-negative bacterium <u>Francisella</u>
(formerly <u>Pasteurella</u>) <u>tularensis</u>, is commonly transmitted
from rodents (particularly rabbits) to man by ticks and
deerflies. However, it is a disease with many focal areas
of high endemicity in different geographic areas, and numerous mammals and arthropods have been implicated in its
transmission. Human infection can also occur following
direct skin contact with infected animals, through ingestion
of contaminated, undercooked animal meat * or contaminated
water, and even through contaminated aerosols. Thus for
tularemia, arthropods are only one of several possible vehicles of transmission.

There are several <u>Borrelia</u> species, all of them Gram-negative
spirochetes, which can be transmitted to humans by body lice
or by soft-bodied ticks. Louse-borne relapsing fever spreads
from person to person in epidemic form under suitable conditions of crowding, poor personal hygiene and social disruption. Its occurrence on a global scale is quite limited at
the present time. However, tick-borne relapsing fever is
enzootic in certain geographic areas (such as the western
United States) and can occur in humans when they intrude
into a natural cycle of animal infection (hunters, for
example).

AN ECOLOGICAL PERSPECTIVE ON INFECTIOUS DISEASES

It should be clear by now that the frequency and distribution
of human infectious diseases can be usefully approached from
a more general ecological perspective. Certain basic questions will usually be pertinent:

-what infectious diseases are unusually frequent (or rare)
 in specific geographic areas or population groups?

-how is the reported frequency of infectious diseases affected by factors such as the route of acquisition, the range
 of hosts infected, the prevalence of the organism in soil,
 and the role of vectors in transmission of disease to humans?

* Moses, in Leviticus, Chapter II, verse 7, proscribes the
eating of rabbit meat because it is "unclean."

-what environmental factors and patterns of human behavior directly contribute to the reported frequency of these diseases?

-what are the implications of these environmental and social factors for infectious disease prevention and/or control?

Table 1 outlines some important factors which may contribute to the frequency of infections. This table, which is presented only as a partial outline of factors potentially involved, should be kept in mind whenever you are considering the range of factors which may enhance or reduce the transmission of bacterial and viral agents. It will be a useful complement to the schematic model of transmission and acquisition of specific infections. You may wish to modify this table for your own future use.

TABLE 1
SOME FACTORS AFFECTING THE FREQUENCY OF HUMAN INFECTIONS

Environmental Factors

geography (terrain, climate, etc.)
animal species (numbers, habits, habitats, etc.)
arthropod species (numbers, habits, etc.)
prevalence and distribution of organisms in soil
type and availability of common food/water sources
man-made environmental changes (dams, etc.)

Social Factors

dwelling arrangements
type and use of domestic animals and pets
usual sources and preparation of food/water
disposition of human excreta
occupational activities and routine habits
beliefs, traditions, customs, taboos, etc.
availability and use of health/medical services
social disruption (earthquake, famine, war, migration)
level of group immunity

THAILAND: AN EXAMPLE

Now examine some statistics reported by the Ministry of
Health in Thailand for the year 1971 (Tables 2 and 3).

TABLE 2

THAILAND: TEN LEADING KNOWN CAUSES OF DEATH, 1971

CAUSE	RATE PER 100,000
Respiratory infections (all forms excluding TB)	34.2
Accidents, poisoning, violence	27.3
Tuberculosis (all forms)	20.8
Diarrheal diseases, typhoid, dysentery	20.4
Diseases of the heart	20.2
Malaria	12.5
Malignant neoplasms	12.4
Diseases of newborns	9.9
Nutritional deficiencies	9.1
Diseases of pregnancy, childbirth, puerperium	7.2

TABLE 3

THAILAND: REPORTED DEATH RATES, 1971

CAUSE	RATE PER 100,000
Ten leading known causes of death, inclusive	171.0
Senility without mention of psychosis	112.8
Symptoms and other ill-defined conditions	266.5
All causes	644.7

III/3, p. 21

Infectious diseases are prominent among these leading reported causes of death, but since over 50% of the reported crude death rate (379.3/100,000 out of 644.7/100,000) is due to "senility," "symptoms," and "other-ill-defined conditions" (none of which are very convincing diagnostic categories), it is hard to know how far to trust the entire set of data. Also remember that these are statistics on death rates and not on incidence or prevalence of specific diseases.

Nevertheless, four of the ten leading causes of death are infections (respiratory infections, TB, diarrheal disease and malaria). Further, many diseases of newborns and many diseases of pregnancy and childbirth are likely to be caused by infectious agents (in a developing country most of the population usually lives in rural areas and the great majority of childbirths occur in the home, in a relatively unsanitary environment). Deaths due to "nutritional deficiencies" are also likely to involve infection as a predominant or contributing factor: whenever childhood malnutrition is prevalent, synergy between infection and malnutrition is a common occurrence. Deaths due to "diseases of the heart" also probably include many patients with advanced rheumatic valvular disease, the end result of an untreated streptococcal infection sometime in the past.

It seems appropriate to conclude that in Thailand:

-tuberculosis and malaria are major national health
 problems

-poor sanitation is an important factor in the high
 death rate from diarrheal diseases

-infectious diseases are a major problem in maternal and
 child health services.

As is usually the case, however, these data on leading causes
of death give an incomplete and misleading picture of the
actual situation with regard to the frequency and community
impact of infectious diseases. Thailand has many other
severe infectious disease problems, including:

-several hundred human deaths from rabies each year (one
 of the highest rabies death rates in the world), due
 to extensive rabies infection of dogs (domestic and
 stray) as well as field rodents, plus frequent human-
 animal contact in farming and forestry;

-recurrent severe outbreaks of dengue hemorrhagic fever
 and Japanese B encephalitis, both caused by arboviruses
 transmitted to humans by mosquitoes;

-tens of thousands of patients with leprosy, a chronic,
 debilitating, socially disruptive and sometimes contagious
 infection;

-recurrent focal cholera epidemics, of minor significance
 in recent years, but always a threat of becoming major
 epidemics because of problems in community sanitation
 and water supplies.

While reported disease-specific death rates may provide a
crude picture of the community impact of certain infections,
much additional information is usually necessary to obtain
a full picture of how infections affect persons in a particular geographic and sociocultural setting. If you were
being assigned to Thailand by the Peace Corps, for example,
you would probably also want to read up on the following
infections (any of which could be a very real threat to
your health): amebiasis, eosinophilic meningitis, scrub
typhus, trichinosis, filariasis, hookworm, and others.
You would probably also be specifically interested in which
diseases were preventable (and how), where you would be at

greatest risk for which infections, how would you recognize
the early manifestations of these diseases, and how (and how
successfully) each of these diseases can be treated. In fact,
in any inquiry regarding the occurrence of infectious
diseases in a foreign setting, one of the best ways to
formulate questions about the risk of infection, the likely
vehicles of transmission and possible means of control and
prevention, is to imagine that you personally are there:
what aspects of the environment, what patterns of social
behavior, and what actions on your own part will enhance or
reduce the likelihood of infection?

Exercise

Imagine that you have been assigned to Thailand for two years, working in public health activities in a rural area. You are particularly anxious not to contract typhoid or rabies. Write in the blank spaces below the letters of those preventive activities in the right-hand column which you think will be most important for you to avoid these two diseases:

DISEASE   PREVENTIVE MEASURES

1) Rabies _____   A) Screen your kitchen

2) Typhoid _____   B) Get immunization(s)

                                           C) Boil all water

                                           D) Take prophylactic anti-
                                                 biotics

                                           E) Avoid raw foods

                                           F) Keep no pets

                                           G) Get rapid care for any
                                                 animal bites

                                           H) Use a proper latrine

SUGGESTED RESPONSES:

1) Rabies   _B,G_

2) Typhoid   _A, B, C, E. H_

Neither disease requires arthropod vectors, although flies
can serve as vehicles of transmission for typhoid bacteria
by carrying them externally from a contaminated site to a
food or water supply. Putting up kitchen screens and
keeping down the population of flies may therefore be very
helpful, but in many rural areas is not feasible. Proper
disposal of human feces is more important. For rabies,
not keeping pets would be little help in Thailand. There
are many stray dogs, and rabies is an extensive zoonosis.
In such a locale where the risk of exposure is high, pre-
exposure immunization is definitely warranted. Rabies immunization is 70-80% effective, using an initial three-dose
series over six months, followed by boosters every 1-2 years
(the ".take" of these immunizations can be monitored by antibody
levels, and the immunization series repeated if necessary).
Following the bite of a suspected or possibly rabid animal,
rapid treatment is indicated. Depending on the
circumstances, this may involve passive immunization with
anti-rabies serum and/or a full course of rabies vaccine.
For typhoid, vaccination is not particularly effective but
should be done. Also, boiling or chlorinating water is
important, as well as avoiding raw foods, especially fruits
and vegetables which may have recently been washed in dirty
water, or any raw food prepared in an unsanitary kitchen
(have you ever examined the kitchen in a restaurant where
you are eating?) . There are no effective prophylactic
antibotics for either disease. Using a proper latrine may
not help you avoid typhoid, but if everyone in the community
did the same, the transmission of typhoid would be sharply
reduced.

Indicate on Figure 4 (rabies) those points in the schematic model where preventive measures would be likely to take effect. Show this by drawing arrows from the specific preventive measure(s) you would suggest to the intervention point on the diagram below:

FIGURE 4

PREVENTION OF RABIES

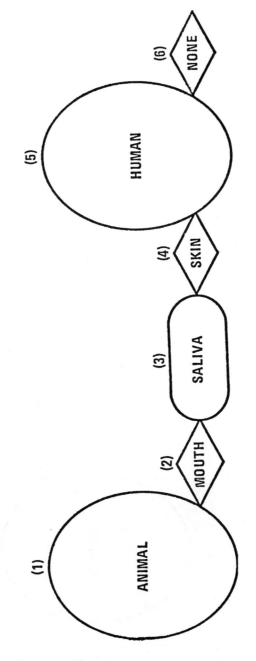

FIGURE 4 (ANSWER)
PREVENTION OF RABIES

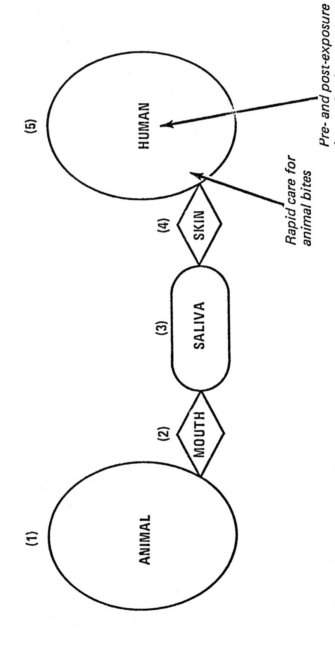

Exercise

Indicate on Figure 5 (typhoid) those points in the schematic model where preventive measures would be likely to take effect. Show this by drawing arrows from the specific preventive measure(s) you would suggest to the intervention point on the diagram below.

FIGURE 5

PREVENTION OF TYPHOID

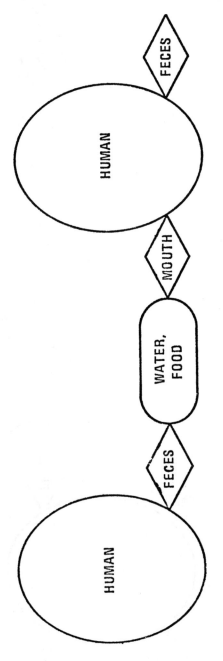

III/3, p. 29

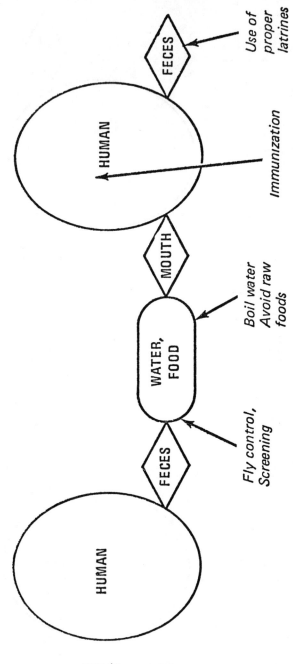

FIGURE 5 (ANSWER)

PREVENTION OF TYPHOID

III/3, p. 30

Of the following five bacterial and viral diseases (all of them already mentioned in this unit), some are relatively frequent in Thailand and some are relatively infrequent. Check below whether you think each disease is relatively frequent or infrequent in Thailand, and give a brief statement of your reason(s) for its relative frequency/ infrequency:

DISEASE	FREQUENT	INFREQUENT	WHY
1. Diphtheria	—	—	_____
2. Leptospirosis	—	—	_____
3. Tetanus	—	—	_____
4. Poliomyelitis	—	—	_____
5. Smallpox	—	—	_____

DISEASE	FREQUENT	INFREQUENT	WHY
1. Diphtheria	X		*Inadequate levels of immunization*
2. Leptospirosis	X		*High exposure to a prevalent zoonosis; no adequate immunization available*
3. Tetanus	X		*Inadequate levels of immunization; nonsterile childbirths (high risk); frequent exposure to soil.*
4. Poliomyelitis		X	*Frequent childhood exposure with mild infections and "natural" immunization*
5. Smallpox		X	*Adequate vaccination levels; disease not endemic; luck.*

INFLUENZA AND SMALLPOX COMPARED

Recent national concern for the possibility of a "swine flu" epidemic in the United States provides an instructive opportunity to consider some of the major factors involved in the occurrence of a widespread infection. Influenza virus spreads readily from person to person by the respiratory route; periodic antigenic shifts in the composition of the virus require ongoing efforts to immunize the general opulation against the current virus; there is no effective anti-influenza therapy; and there are no important animal hosts or vectors which can be attacked as a means for controlling influenza.

Smallpox is also a viral illness transmitted from person to person, usually via the respiratory route; it does not involve animal hosts or vectors; and there is no effective therapy on a community-wide scale. However, smallpox, unlike influenza, has recently been virtually eradicated on a worldwide basis.

There are several important differences between these two viral diseases, influenza and smallpox, in terms of their susceptibility to prevention as major infectious disease problems. These differences include the following:

1. Smallpox infection confers immunity for life. Influenza infection does not, due to periodic antigenic shifts in viral composition.

2. Because of the stability of viral antigens, smallpox vaccination provides effective immunity against viral infection. For influenza, repeated and updated immunization is required for current protection.

3. Persons with inapparent or mild influenza infection may not be recognized but are still contagious to others. With smallpox, infected persons have systemic infections with significant skin involvement, and are more readily identified as "cases" to be avoided either by formal quarantine or by social avoidance.

4. Smallpox has behaved in recent years as a fairly stable endemic disease, largely confined to specific geographic areas and rapidly being eradicated by WHO control efforts. Influenza occurs as an annual worldwide epidemic of varying severity, and is not amenable to eradication because of periodic antigenic shifts.

One important topic related to prevention and control (but not yet discussed) is the general level of immunity to specific infections within a particular population group. Obviously, if an entire population is completely immune to an infection, human infection will not occur.

Conversely, absent or unusually low levels of immunity may allow epidemic spread of diseases which otherwise would have minor community impact. Island communities (in the Aleutians, for example, or in the South Pacific) have often experienced explosive epidemics of measles, mumps, influenza, or other respiratory viruses which had been absent from these communities for many years and which spread rapidly from person to person by close contact. There is no "magic number" which represents the precise level of population immunity (or "herd immunity") which is sufficient to prevent the rapid spread of communicable diseases. For many respiratory viruses, it is generally felt that if 70-80% of a community is immune, the possibility of epidemic spread is small.

Check those diseases for which adequate (safe and effective) immunizations are now available:

	YES	NO
Cholera	_____	_____
Diphtheria	_____	_____
Measles	_____	_____
Poliomyelitis	_____	_____
Tetanus	_____	_____

	YES	NO
Cholera		X
Diphtheria	X	
Measles	X	
Poliomyelitis	X	
Tetanus	X	

Cholera vaccine (made from killed vibrios) is available, but is generally only 70-80% effective and lasts only for six months or less. Frequent re-vaccination of entire communities is extremely difficult. Diphtheria toxoid (made from inactivated toxin) is effective if given repeatedly (three basic immunizations in the first year of life, with booster doses one and four years later, then every 5-10 years). Measles vaccine (a live attenuated virus preparation) is probably effective for life after a single dose. Polio immunization is generally effective when given as a basic childhood series (using oral trivalent live attentuated virus). Tetanus toxoid is routinely given on the same schedule as diphtheria toxoid (see above). In previously immunized adults, additional tetanus boosters are protective for up to 10 years. In developing countries where neonatal tetanus is a major concern, two doses of tetanus toxoid to pregnant women are dramatically effective in reducing the incidence of tetanus among newborns, and even a single dose offers substantial protection.

In addition to immunization provided by injections and oral vaccines, "natural" immunization is also an important phenomenon and a major contributor to population immunity. Certain infections which may occur frequently in childhood (such as polio virus infection under relatively unsanitary conditions in certain countries) may cause inapparent or mild disease in children but can confer immunity for life.

CONCLUSION

This brief overview of bacterial and viral infections has been intended primarily to give you a conceptual framework and to stimulate questions for your further investigation, as your time and interest permit. Remember that the schematic model of disease transmission is only a starting point, and its major use in this unit has been to help you think about questions such as the following:

A. For what **bacterial** and **viral** diseases does food or water served as a usual vehicle of transmission?

    1) _____

    2) _____

    3) _____

    4) _____

B. What is the usual reservoir of infection (human vs. animal) for the following:

DISEASE	USUAL RESERVOIR	
	ANIMAL	HUMAN
1. Typhoid	_____	_____
2. Smallpox	_____	_____
3. Diphtheria	_____	_____
4. Leprosy	_____	_____
5. Tularemia	_____	_____

SUGGESTED RESPONSES

A. 1) *typhoid*
    2) *cholera*
    3) *salmonellosis (non-typhoid)*
    4) *polio*

B. DISEASE

DISEASE	USUAL RESERVOIR	
	HUMAN	ANIMAL
Typhoid	X	
Smallpox	X	
Diphtheria	X	
Leprosy	X	
Tularemia		X

USEFUL REFERENCES

1) Benenson, A.S. Control of Communicable Diseases in Man, APHA, 1975 (12th Edition)

2) Hoeprich, Paul (editor). Infectious Diseases, Harper and Row, 1972

UNIT III/4: PARASITIC DISEASES I. SCHISTOSOMIASIS

BY

MICHAEL M. STEWART, M.D., M.P.H.
RICHARD H. MORROW JR., M.D.

CONTENTS

OBJECTIVES

This instructional unit introduces the broad subject of
human parasitic diseases through detailed examination of
one disease, schistosomiasis. The major emphases are: the
ecological determinants of transmission, pathogenesis, the
spectrum of human illness, the effects of disease on human
communities, and possible methods of control.

At the completion of this unit, you will be able to:

1. Illustrate the interrelationships of the major components
in the schistosome life cycle by drawing a schematic summary
diagram;

2. Indicate on this diagram how ecological factors and
human behavior affect the schistosome life cycle;

3. Identify the points in the life cycle where different
methods of intervention can interrupt transmission of
schistosomiasis.

SCHISTOSOMIASIS - THE DISEASE AND ITS SETTING

AN ILLUSTRATIVE CASE

A 22-year old man was admitted to Gulu Hospital in January
1975 with the chief complaint of vomiting blood. The
patient's health had been generally good until the previous
month, when he began to develop nausea and a sense of
abdominal fullness. Two days before hospital admission he
abruptly vomited several cupfuls of dark red-black material.
This continued intermittently for several hours and he became
sweaty, light-headed and very weak. Unable to walk, he was
brought to the hospital by his family.

III/4, p. 2

To a clinician, this brief history would immeditately suggest several important diagnostic possibilities. Based on your own medical school experience to date, list the two most likely diagnostic possibilities if this patient had been seen in the emergency room of your university hospital:

1.

2.

Your list should have included "ruptured esophageal varices" and "bleeding peptic ulcer" as possible causes of sudden and severe upper gastrointestinal bleeding. (There are also many other less frequent causes). However, the frequency of different diseases which cause esophageal varices may vary with the geographic setting. In Boston, bleeding varices (particularly in older men) would most often be due to alcoholic cirrhosis of the liver with secondary portal hypertension. In India, where alcoholic cirrhosis is rare, esophageal varices occur frequently in patients with advanced cirrhosis or portal fibrosis of unknown cause.

The patient described above lived in a small village in the West Nile district of Uganda, in East Africa, and the underlying cause of his life-threatening hemorrhage was an advanced stage of schistosomiasis* due to infection with the human parasite Schistosoma mansoni. This disease, which affects some 250-300 million people throughout the world, causes many different clinical problems. In the case presented, large numbers of schistosome eggs had been lodged in the patient's liver for many years, eventually leading to extensive fibrosis and the development of portal hypertension with esophageal varices. The patient's dramatic episode of bleeding resulted from variceal rupture, and the patient died in the hospital. No autopsy was performed.

This case is a dramatic example of the terminal stage of schistosomiasis, one of the most important human parasitic

---

* Schistosomiasis is sometimes referred to, particularly in the older literature, as Bilharziasis, after Theodor Bilharz, the discoverer of the schistosome worm in 1862.

diseases (or parasitoses). In many areas of the tropics and subtropics, this is a common disease with a wide spectrum of symptoms ranging from very mild to severe. Its medical and social consequences are considerable. The disease is maintained in human populations through direct involvement of humans in the life cyle of the schistosome parasite. Infection is acquired by direct skin contact with water contaminated by a motile stage of the parasite which has been released from infected snails. Continued transmission is made possible by the persisting discharge of egg-containing human excreta into fresh water where the presence of suitable snails permits continued multiplication of the parasite.

Geographically, schistosomiasis is found in most countries of Africa, in limited areas of the Near East, in several heavily populated Asian countries (China, Taiwan, the Philippines), and, in the western hemisphere, in northeast Brazil, Surinam, Venezuela and several Caribbean islands. Because schistosomiasis is not transmitted within the United States, American physicians see only imported cases (patients whose infections have been acquired abroad), and they are therefore generally unfamiliar with the clinical spectrum of schistosomiasis, as well as with its epidemiologic patterns. However, since more than 200 million people in the world have schistosomiasis, anyone interested in international health must view this disease as a major problem. Several international agencies have made it a high priority, and the World Health Organization has recently included schistosomiasis as one of six infectious diseases as the targets of a 10-year research and control program. (The other diseases are filariasis, leishmaniasis, malaria, trypanosomiasis, and leprosy).

Schistosomiasis is also one of the most rapidly
increasing major parasitic disease problems in the
world. Ironically, this increase is largely the direct
result of man-made environmental alterations carried out
in order to improve human welfare. Dams, irrigation
schemes, and agricultural techniques utilized to enhance
economic productivity have led to a rapid increase and
spread of those snails involved in schistosomiasis
transmission in many parts of Asia, Africa and Latin
America. These programs, promoted in the name of economic
development, often provide ideal conditions for snail
proliferation and simultaneously attract large new human
communities to these same areas. This rapid increase in
both snail and human populations leads to a geometric
increase in opportunities for parasite transmission.
In the past decade, schistosomiasis has become a major,
acute disease problem, perhaps most dramatically
documented in Ghana as a result of the construction of
the Volta Dam, and in Egypt with the development of Lake
Nasser.

Preassessment

At this point, please list the major questions about schistosomiasis which you would like to have answered by the end of this instructional unit (list three to five questions):

1.

2.

3.

4.

5.

SUGGESTED QUESTIONS

The questions which you have listed will obviously depend on your current knowledge of epidemiology, parasitology (schistosomiasis in particular), public health, preventive medicine and clinical medicine. This instructional unit is necessarily limited in scope, and will deal primarily with the questions below. It is hoped that at least some of yours are included.

What is the life cycle of the schistosome parasite and how is it transmitted?

What environmental and behavioral factors facilitate transmission?

How does the parasite cause human disease?

What are the effects of schistosomiasis on human populations?

How can schistosomiasis be controlled?

This unit will not provide details on the clinical management or chemotherapy of schistosomiasis. If any of your major questions have not been answered at the end of this unit, a list of suggested further reading is also supplied. You may wish to keep in mind the following underlying concepts as you progress through the remainder of the unit:

UNDERLYING CONCEPTS

The specific cause of a particular clinical syndrome may vary with the geographic location. What is unusual in one location may be common elsewhere.

A clinician should think as an epidemiologist, and should always consider those aspects of time-place-person which may have put a patient at risk of acquiring particular diseases.

THE PATIENT'S COMMUNITY

The village in which this young Ugandan man lived is located in a low swampy area on the western shore of the Nile River in East Central Africa. The village way of life has changed little for many generations, and people survive primarily by a combination of simple farming, with grain as the basic crop, and fishing in the Nile for their major protein source. Houses are made of wood and mud with thatched roofs and floors of pounded clay. Family groups are large, frequently including grandparents, relatives and many children. Most married women have six to ten pregnancies, with four or five surviving children. The temperature is above 70 degrees F. all year and clothing is simple. Heavy rains occur during two seasons, September-November and April-May, but water for household purposes is abundant all year through proximity to the fresh-water river. Domestic animals are not regularly used as beasts of burden, and most families keep only a few chickens. There are no toilets; latrines are few and their use is irregular. People commonly defecate and urinate into or near the river. Untreated river water is used for almost all household purposes. Primary school education is available, but most of the village adults are currently illiterate. No Western-style medical care services are available in the village, and the patient described above had to be transported 80 miles by bus to reach Gulu Hospital.

From this description of the patient's community,
which four of the eight features of village life
listed belov do you think are particularly
important in helping to maintain schistosomiasis as
an _endemic_ (always present) disease in this village?
(Check the appropriate answers).

_____1. Use of river water for most domestic purposes

_____2. Long distance to the nearest hospital

_____3. Proximity of the village to a fresh-water river

_____4. Houses made of wood and thatched roofs

_____5. Large family groups

_____6. Fishing as a major occupation

_____7. Defecation and urination near the river

_____8. Widespread adult illiteracy

__X__ 1. Use of river water for most domestic purposes

_____ 2. Long distance to the nearest hospital

__X__ 3. Proximity of the village to a fresh-water river

_____ 4. Houses made of wood and thatched roofs

_____ 5. Large family groups

__X__ 6. Fishing as a major occupation

__X__ 7. Defecation and urination near the river

_____ 8. Widespread adult illiteracy

In order for schistosomiasis to be maintained as an endemic infection in any community, the cycle of transmission from human to snail to human must be continued. Although you may not yet understand the details of this transmission cycle, your knowledge that it involves human contact with water containing motile parasitic forms released from infected snails should have helped you to identify the factors facilitating transmission as checked above.

Appreciating the close relationship of human populations to water is essential in understanding epidemiological patterns of schistosomiasis. In this particular Ugandan village (and in many others like it around the world), close contact with river water is inevitable. Everyone uses the river for bathing, for washing clothes, and for drinking. Even in the rainy season, it is easier to obtain river water than rain water for drinking, and the river water is simply collected into pots for settling before use. The water is not boiled, and no chemicals are used. In hotter weather, everyone bathes several times daily. Because of obvious hazards, infants and young children are allowed only limited access to the river, but adolescents and young adults spend much time with the older village men in fishing, and also with women in drawing water and helping with domestic washing. The water's edge is a natural place for community socialization, as well as for village occupations. Water is also a necessity for animals, both domestic and wild.

In many tropical areas, this degree of close personal contact with water is a necessary facet of village life. Water supplies are central to a community's survival, and water may therefore be directly or indirectly involved in many of a community's major health and disease problems.

In addition to schistosomiasis, what other diseases and health hazards do you think are likely to affect the residents of an African village as a direct result of proximity to water or habits of water use? Try to name three:

1.

2.

3.

SUGGESTED RESPONSES

This question goes beyond the immediate scope of this instructional unit, but it is important for you to think of schistosomiasis within a broader context of water-related health hazards:

1. *Bacterial, viral and parasitic diseases caused by ingestion of water polluted with fecal matter (typhoid, polio and amebiasis, for example).*

2. *Diseases carried by insects breeding in water (malaria, onchocerciasis).*

3. *Water-related trauma and accidents.*

UNDERLYING CONCEPTS

Village life in tropical areas often involves close contact with one predominant water source.

Water sources may be directly associated with a variety of health hazards.

COMMUNITY IMPACT OF SCHISTOSOMIASIS

You now have a rough mental picture of a "typical" village
in which continued transmission of <u>Schistosoma mansoni</u> is
supported by the right combination of environmental
circumstances and human habits. It is important at this
point to consider the various ways in which this chronic
disease can affect a community and how this community
impact could be measured. The basic concepts and definitions
for assessment of a community's health status are given in
Unit II/1, Assessment of Health Problems and Resources: Concepts.

What specific types of information would be most useful in
determining the impact of <u>Schistosoma mansoni</u> in an African
village? (List at least four items).

1.

2.

3.

4.

There are several types of epidemiological information about schistosomiasis that would be relevant, such as incidence, prevalence, intensity of infection, chronicity and severity of disease, and mortality due to schistosomiasis. Furthermore, age-specific incidence, prevalence and mortality rates, as well as how and to what extent schistosomiasis interferes with the routine conduct of daily village affairs (work productivity, child-rearing, etc.), would be essential information in assessing the impact on community life.

Unfortunately, detailed epidemiological information is rarely available in African villages. Even basic vital statistics are not routinely kept, and the following are only rough current estimates for western Uganda:

Crude Birth Rate: 55/1000 per year
Crude Death Rate: 25/1000 per year
Infant Death Rate: 150/1000 live births per year
Childhood Death Rate (ages 1-4):   120/1000 per year

Disease-specific prevalence data for Uganda are unknown, but a special study conducted in the patient's village found that everyone over the age of 10 was infected with S. mansoni. Many young adults die after developing large swollen abdomens, and children often suffer from (and occasionally die with) bloody diarrhea. There are many other serious diseases (malaria, hookworm, typhoid, tuberculosis), but villagers do not directly associate disease with water contact or with their own habits of water use.

UNDERLYING CONCEPTS

Basic information on the community impact of schistosomiasis is rarely available in rural areas.

In many areas of the world, several different infectious diseases are endemic. It is often difficult to assess the community impact of these diseases, taken either separately or together.

THE CHAIN OF EVENTS IN HUMAN INFECTION

THE LIFE CYCLE OF SCHISTOSOMES

The young Ugandan patient with gastrointestinal bleeding had advanced liver disease due to chronic infection with <u>Schistosoma mansoni</u>. There are three major species of schistosomes which infect humans:

<u>Schistosoma mansoni</u>, <u>Schistosoma japonicum</u> and <u>Schistosoma hematobium</u>. All three schistosomes have essentially the same life cycle, which is simple in outline, but biologically rather complex. (See Unit III/5 for the biological classification of schistosomes and other parasites). Note in Figure 1 that there are four essential components in the schistosome life cycle.

1. snails

2. humans

3. the schistosome parasite

4. water

Reproduction by the parasite occurs within both human and snail hosts. Sexual reproduction occurs within the infected human host, called the <u>definitive host</u> (harboring sexually mature adult parasites), with production of large numbers of eggs. Within the snail host, which is termed an <u>intermediate host</u> (harboring asexual stages of the parasite), two stages of asexual reproduction occur.

The geographic distribution of a particular schistosome species is primarily dependent upon the distribution of a particular snail species: there is a high degree of specificity in the species of snail in which a given

FIGURE 1

BASIC LIFE CYCLE OF SCHISTOSOMES

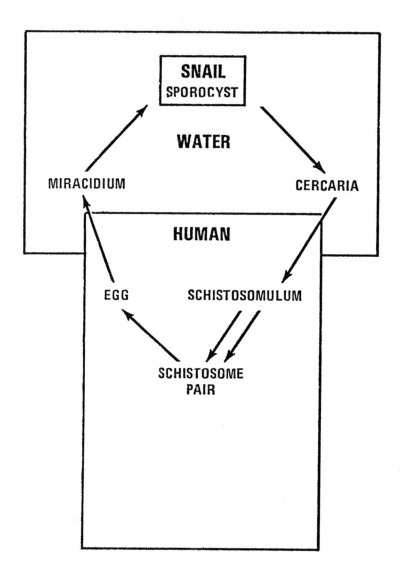

schistosome can develop. S. hematobium, limited to Africa and the Middle East, can develop only in certain snail species which belong to the genera Bulinus and Physopsis. S. mansoni, found in Africa and the Middle East and also in South America and the Caribbean, requires snails of the Biomphalaria genus for its development. S. japonicum, which is confined to the Far East, can develop only in snails of the Oncomelania genus. All of the above snails are fresh water species, and all are microherbivores (scavengers of vegetative debris). The Biomphalaria and Bulinus groups are air-breathing water snails, are hermaphrodites, and can live under field conditions (out of water) for periods up to one year. Oncomelania snails have gills and are amphibious. They have separate sexes and have a life span up to five years. Infection with schistosomiasis is harder on the snail than it is on humans; infected snails generally have shortened life spans and decreased fertility.

It should be noted that certain animals also can become involved in the schistosome life cycle in the same way that humans do. For S. mansoni and S. hematobium, infection of small numbers of monkeys, baboons and rodents is not of major epidemiological significance. However, S. Japonicum infects a wide variety of mammals other than humans (cattle, pigs, horses, water buffalo, cats, dogs, rats, goats, etc.). These animals are known as reservoir hosts (non-human hosts which harbor sexually mature adult parasites), and are important because they shed large numbers of schistosome eggs into the environment in their excreta. These schistosome eggs can eventually produce parasite forms which are infective both for humans and other animals. There are areas of the world in which animal infections are the predominant problem. In Taiwan, for example, one species of S. japonicum is strictly zoonotic, with non-human animals as the definitive host for this species, and with no involvement of humans.

The details of the schistosome life cycle can be summarized as follows, starting with the reproductive adult schistosome pairs in the human host:

Fertilized eggs are excreted in human urine or feces. These eggs hatch soon after entering fresh water under the proper conditions of osmolality, light and warmth. Each egg releases a free-swimming larval form called a _miracidium_, which has a life span of less than 24 hours. These motile miracidia seek out and penetrate certain species of aquatic snails, which they infect and utilize as intermediate hosts. Within a snail, the miracidium develops into a larval stage called a _mother sporocyst_. Each mother sporocyst in turn gives rise to multiple _daughter sporocysts_, each of which by asexual budding produces thousands of further larval forms called _cercariae_. Five to six weeks after the initial penetration of a snail by a miracidium, free-swimming fork-tailed cercariae begin to be shed by the snail into surrounding fresh water. Shedding of cercariae on a daily basis (up to 1000/day for _S. hematobium_ and _S. mansoni_) continues for the life of the snail.

All cercariae produced from one miracidium are of the same sex, and all cercariae, while morphologically similar, are genetically destined to develop into either male or female schistosomes. Like miracidia, cercariae are short-lived. Upon contacting human skin, the cercariae drop their tails and penetrate to the subdermal capillaries and lymphatics, becoming _schistosomula_ (young schistosomes). These invading schistosomula then progress through the human venous circulation to the lungs, through the pulmonary capillary bed, and in a manner not entirely understood, into the intrahepatic portal venules. Here schistosomula mature into adult schistosomes, meet their mates, and make their way to their final distination. _S. hematobium_ has a poorly understood _tropism_ (tissue orientation) for the vesical (urinary bladder) venous system, while _S. mansoni_ and _S. japonicum_ settle primarily in the mesenteric (intestinal) venous system. Within the various venous plexuses, these adult schistosomes mate, and after a few weeks female schistosomes begin depositing eggs. Adult worm pairs may remain together for many years, producing hundreds of eggs each day.

The adult schistosomes by themselves cause no major problem for humans. Adult worms do not obstruct venous drainage, nor do they usually produce a significant inflammatory response. However, eggs produced by these worm pairs provoke a considerable inflammatory response. Many eggs work their way into the lumen of the intestine and the urinary bladder, often accompanied by inflammatory cells and small amounts of local hemorrhage. Other eggs become lodged in the walls of involved viscera, with gradual development of inflammatory foci around them (granulomata) and fibrosis. With S. mansoni and S. japonicum, some schistosome eggs are swept back via the portal circulation into the periportal areas of the liver. In heavy infections, these eggs initiate an inflammatory reaction which may eventually lead to extensive periportal fibrosis. Some eggs may also occasionally reach the caval and vertebral venous systems and lodge in the lungs, spinal cord or other organs.

A Quick Review

1. When humans are infected with schistosomiasis, which stage of the schistosome parasite is the primary cause of human disease?

    (a) _____ miracidium
    (b) _____ cercaria
    (c) _____ schistosomulum
    (d) _____ adult schistosome
    (e) _____ egg

2. In addition to the schistosome parasite in its various stages of development, what are the three other major ecologic components required for continuation of the schistosome life cycle?

    (a)

    (b)

    (c)

1. *Human disease is primarily caused by host reaction to the presence of schistosome <u>EGGS</u> (e) in human tissue.*

2. *(a) <u>WATER</u> as a supporting milieu for development of parasite forms in snails and as a route of transmission for miracidia to snails and for cercariae to human skin.*

(b) <u>HUMANS</u> as definitive hosts (for <u>S. japonicum</u>, other animals may also serve as definitive hosts).

(c) <u>SNAILS</u> as intermediate hosts for schistosome multiplication.

It is important at this point to reemphasize certain aspects of the schistosome life cycle shown in Figure 1 (p. 18) in terms of the risk to humans. One egg produces one <u>miracidium</u>, which infects one <u>snail</u>, resulting in 100,000 or more <u>cercariae</u>. Each infecting cercaria produces one <u>schistosomulum</u>, which matures into one male or female <u>schistosome</u>. Each mating pair of adult schistosomes may produce many hundreds of thousands (millions) of <u>eggs</u> over a period of years.

The production of cercariae in the snail and of eggs in the human are the two stages of great <u>multiplication potential</u> (1 to 10^5 or 10^6 in each). Thus, a relatively low prevalence of infection in snails can result in a high transmission rate in humans, provided that human exposure to contaminated water is maintained.

UNDERLYING CONCEPT

Knowledge of the parasitic life cycle is essential for understanding both the epidemiology and pathophysiology of human schistosomiasis, as well as its treatment and control. This is generally true for human parasitic diseases (See also Unit III/5.)

PATHOGENESIS OF THE DISEASE

The major pathological features of chronic schistosomiasis due to S. mansoni and S. japonicum are extensive granulomatous involvement of the large bowel, periportal fibrosis of the liver, and, with S. hematobium, fibrosis of the urinary bladder and ureters. The critical factor in determining the extent of tissue damage is the number of eggs deposited, which itself is a function of the worm burden (total number of mating worm pairs present), and the length of time during which continuing oviposition (deposition of eggs) has taken place.

A post-mortem examination of the young Ugandan man described above might have revealed the following findings (among others):

. hepatomegaly with portal fibrosis

. prominent splenomegaly with dilated portal and splenic veins

. gross or microscopic evidence of dense periportal fibrosis ("pipestem fibrosis"), as well as multiple hepatic granulomata, some formed around intact S. mansoni eggs or fragments of degenerating eggs

. adult worms (and worm pairs) within the mesenteric veins

. multiple granulomata throughout the intestinal tract, organized around fragments of schistosome eggs.

Schistosomiasis affects humans as a chronic visceral infection. The major impact is seen in the liver, spleen and intestine (S. mansoni and S. japonicum), or in the bladder, ureters and kidneys (S. hematobium). The mechanism of host response to the deposition of eggs is complex, and will not be further considered in detail in this unit.

In addition to upper gastrointestinal bleeding due to ruptured esophageal varices, there are several other major clinical problems which you might expect to encounter in patients with advanced S. mansoni infection. Can you name two?

1.

2.

Some selected examples of other major clinical problems include:

1. Anemia due to several factors, including poor appetite, blood loss and hemolytic anemia related to hypersplenism.

2. Bowel problems such as diarrhea, abdominal pain, hemorrhoids, and rectal prolapse, all due to direct involvement of the bowel wall (particularly the large bowel) in the granulomatous reaction to schistosome eggs.

3. Pulmonary symptoms caused by reaction to eggs which may have embolized to pulmonary vessels (extensive involvement of the pulmonary arterial circulation can occasionally cause right-sided congestive heart failure, or cor pulmonale).

UNDERLYING CONCEPTS

The clinical features of advanced schistosomiasis are directly related to the distribution and numbers of adult worms and the eggs which they produce. The total number of adult schistosomes (or intensity of infection) is directly related to the frequency and intensity of exposure to cercariae.

Many parasitic diseases affect particular organ systems in the course of human infections, and knowledge of the causation of human disease requires knowledge of how parasites invade and establish infections in their human hosts.

THE SPECTRUM OF HUMAN ILLNESS

Up to this point, we have focused on chronic infection with S. mansoni. However, the symptoms, signs and prognosis of all three types of schistosomiasis are extremely variable and depend on the type, intensity and duration of infection. The range of clinical problems seen in schistosomiasis can be classified according to the length of time following initial infection. For example, clinical problems can be correlated with each of the following stages of parasite development in the human host: (1) invasion, (2) maturation, (3) oviposition and (4) persistence.

1. Invasion. As cercariae penetrate human skin, there may be a phase of dermatitis and other allergic symptoms. Signs and symptoms at this stage are usually mild. Dermatitis may also occur if schistosomes which normally infect birds (avian schistosomes) invade humans, causing a condition known as "swimmer's itch." This is seen in the mid-western United States, after contact with fresh water lakes infested with avian schistosomes.

2. Maturation. During the several-week period when schistosomula migrate and mature into adult schistosomes within the portal circulation, a patient may experience mild fever, eosinophilia, and abdominal pain. These symptoms, which precede the beginning of oviposition, probably reflect the systemic effects of an immune response to worm antigens, and they subside spontaneously.

3. Oviposition. As eggs are produced and deposited within venules and work their way into surrounding tissues, severe inflammatory reaction takes place. The exact symptoms depend on the organs involved, the number of eggs, and the extent of inflammation and tissue damage. For example, extensive involvement of the bowel may produce acute dysentery, with severe diarrhea and gastrointestinal blood loss.

4. Persistence. As noted above, chronic infections may cause widespread granulomata and fibrosis, with gradual compromise of involved viscera related to the extent and location of egg deposition.

It must be stressed that repeated infections of persons in endemic areas can cause considerable overlap in these temporal stages of clinical illness. In addition, host immune defenses play an active but as yet incompletely understood role in responding to schistosome infections.

A few brief words on diagnosis are appropriate. In most cases a firm diagnosis of schistosomiasis can be made by demonstration of schistosome eggs in specimens of stool or urine, using relatively simple laboratory techniques. The species of infecting schistosome is readily determined by characteristic features of its eggs, and the intensity of human infection is gauged by quantitative measurement of the number of eggs per volume or weight of excreta. Demonstration of specific organ damage may require a biopsy (for example, of the liver or rectal mucosa). Immunodiagnosis is not presently an efficient or reliable diagnostic tool, although skin tests and serum antibody tests are used for investigative purposes.

TREATMENT

Treatment is quite specialized. There are a number of drugs which have some effect, and adult S. hematobium and S. mansoni worms can be effectively killed by relatively nontoxic drugs. However, these drugs are not recommended for mass chemotherapy. Moreover, therapy does not reverse the fibrotic changes seen in advanced disease, nor does it prevent reinfection in patients who continue to be exposed to infested water sources. At present there is no effective means of immunization against infection.

What medical advice would you offer to a Peace Corps volunteer assigned for two years to an African village where S. mansoni is known to be endemic? (Check all that apply).

_____ 1. Take prophylactic medication.

_____ 2. Boil all drinking water.

_____ 3. Have a checkup yearly.

_____ 4. Avoid direct skin-to-water contact with infested water.

_____ 5. Have a blood test to determine immunity.

*The best answer is to avoid **direct** skin-to-water contact with water sources where snails may exist (#4). This may not be easy, of course, and may mean thinking twice before taking a swim, or venturing out in a small boat.*

Also, and something not previously mentioned, it means avoiding drinking of contaminated water, since cercariae can penetrate the human oropharyngeal mucusa just as they penetrate external human skin. Therefore, boiling all drinking water (#2) is also a good idea, and may prevent other infectious diseases as well. A yearly checkup (#3) might help to identify mild infections and lead to early treatment, if the history and physical examination are thorough and the appropriate laboratory tests are done. However, there is no effective prophylactic drug (#1), nor is there any routine "blood test to determine immunity" (#5). Also, as noted previously, there is no available prophylactic immunization.

Now examine Figure 2. As you will note, it is an extension of Figure 1, expanded to include the ecology of schistosomiasis as it affects humans. The vertical left-hand margin indicates the four general types of problems created for human communities at various stages of the extended life cycle, while the vertical right-hand margin indicates five ways to measure the extent of the problem at each stage. These measurement techniques include: determining the percent of snails infected with schistosomes in a given ecological setting; calculation of the number of free-swimming cercariae in a given volume of fresh water (cercariometry); measurement of the number of schistosome eggs in a given volume or weight of human excreta; identifying the presence of schistosome eggs in human tissue, and also noting the type and extent of tissue damage (morbidity data); and the reporting of disease-specific mortality rates due to schistosomiasis.

FIGURE 2

SCHISTOSOMIASIS AS A COMMUNITY HEALTH PROBLEM*

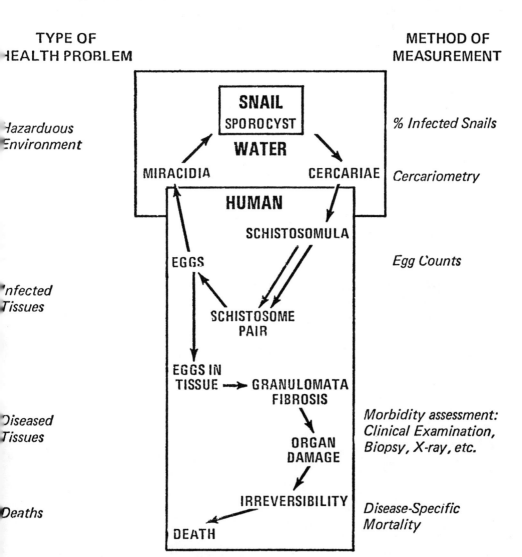

TYPE OF
HEALTH PROBLEM

METHOD OF
MEASUREMENT

Hazarduous
Environment

% Infected Snails

SNAIL
SPOROCYST
WATER

MIRACIDIA   CERCARIAE   Cercariometry

HUMAN

SCHISTOSOMULA

EGGS   Egg Counts

Infected
Tissues

SCHISTOSOME
PAIR

EGGS IN
TISSUE → GRANULOMATA
FIBROSIS

Diseased
Tissues

ORGAN
DAMAGE

Morbidity assessment:
Clinical Examination,
Biopsy, X-ray, etc.

IRREVERSIBILITY

Deaths   Disease-Specific
Mortality

DEATH

* adapted from Kenneth Warren, M.D., with permission

In a conceptual sense, Figure 2 represents a framework for considering the various aspects of schistosomiasis as an endemic community health problem. The important questions are not only: Who has schistosomiasis? or, How many people have schistosomiasis? It is also important to consider the amount of infection per individual, i.e. , the number of worm pairs as reflected by egg counts, the stage of infection, how that stage is measured, and how the pattern of schistosomiasis prevalence is related to local environmental and behavioral factors. Quantitation is a critical step in determining which phase of the transmission cycle may be most effectively attacked.

UNDERLYING CONCEPTS

The key variables in understanding the type of human illness caused by schistosomiasis are the schistosome species, and the location and severity of reaction to the presence of eggs in human tissues.

Immunization is not effective. Drug therapy is not as effective as prevention of exposure.

CONTROL OF SCHISTOSOMIASIS

ECOLOGICAL DETERMINANTS

Applying your understanding of Figures 1 (page 18) and 2 (page 31), list four possible methods for controlling the transmission of schistosomiasis:

1.

2.

3.

4.

SUGGESTED RESPONSES

Any measure which effectively interrupts the life cycle of schistosomes will be an important control measure (eliminating the human population, however, is <u>not</u> considered practical). Measures which you might have considered include the following:

1. _Prevent schistosome eggs from reaching water.*_
2. _Prevent miracidia from infecting snails._
3. _Control (or eliminate) the snail population._
4. _Prevent cercariae from contacting human skin._
5. _Prevent schistosomula from maturing into adult schistosomes within humans._
6. _Prevent adult schistosomes from producing eggs._

CONTROL MEASURES

A sensible approach to the control of <u>S. mansoni</u> would be to attempt to prevent the contamination of fresh water sources with human feces containing schistosome eggs (recall here the "indiscriminate defecation" in the Ugandan village). The introduction of an adequate privy or latrine system, or even adherence to simple instructions about where to defecate, would theoretically be sufficient to stop further disease transmission. However, the "sanitary approach" has generally not proven an effective control measure. For one thing, sanitary conveniences (even simple pit latrines) are relatively costly. In many areas of the world, total governmental and personal expenditures on health services are less than U.S. $5 per person per year, and a pit latrine

---

* Special problems are presented by the contamination of human water sources by the excreta of non-human animals infected with <u>S. japonicum</u>. These problems are not discussed in this unit.

may cost many times that amount. In addition, pit latrines (particularly in wet tropical areas) may be esthestically unacceptable for obvious reasons. They also are hazardous for small children, particularly when dug deeply. Most societies have certain rules concerning defecation, but virtually nowhere has an effective privy system been established without strong external pressure from a governmental authority.

Quantitative considerations are also important. A single schistosome egg, producing one miracidium, may give rise to 100,000 cercariae within a few months. Given this multiplication potential, and assuming the presence of an appropriate number and type of fresh water snails, a sanitation system would have to be virtually perfect to prevent proliferation of schistosomes. One child with urgent misplaced defecation could support disease transmission to an entire village, if frequent human exposure to infested water continued.

The second critical quantitative factor is that adult worm pairs continue to produce eggs for many years. Any sanitary system designed to prevent schistosomiasis must thus be not only comprehensive but also durable over long periods of time.

Now try to identify at least two lines of argument, other than cost, which might be advanced by African villagers against attempts to install privies as a means of schistosomiasis control:

1.

2.

These answers are not based on specific village circumstances, but rather on the general experience of the authors in less developed countries:

1. Villagers do not believe that human feces or urine have anything to do with disease.

2. Defecation and urination are personal affairs, not to be regulated by any authority.

3. Defecation into fresh water is "cleaner" than into a privy.

4. Privies breed flies and mosquitoes, which are known to cause disease.

5. Animals do not use privies, so why should humans?

The major point here is that measures which may appear rational from a sanitary engineering perspective may appear irrational (or at least unwarranted) within a specific local society and culture.

A second general method of control would be to prevent contact between the human population and infested (contaminated) water. This method would require the availability of abundant purified water for daily use, and would rely heavily on advice to the local populace to avoid direct contact with polluted natural water sources in order to avoid infection. Again, the cost of such a clean water system is usually prohibitive in rural tropical areas with low density populations. In some pilot projects, abundant purified water has been made available, but the lure of bathing in cool natural water on a hot day may prove irresistible, particularly since river banks, ponds and springs are natural places for social gatherings. The provision of a "safe" water source should be viewed as a necessary but not a sufficient condition for controlling schistosomiasis.

Much recent effort has been focused on the destruction or reduction of snails, chiefly by use of chemical poisons, since without the right numbers and types of snails to serve as intermediate hosts, transmission will cease. The various snails involved in the life cycle of each of the three schistosomes prosper in a wide variety of ecological settings, and control measures must be targeted to suit local conditions. As noted previously, dams and other development schemes have directly contributed to snail proliferation.

In general, there are four types of ecological settings to be considered for the application of snail control measures:

- rivers and streams with running water

- ponds and swamps with relatively stagnant water

- large lakes (both natural and impounded) with large surface areas and shifting shorelines

- large-scale irrigation systems where water inflow can be intentionally regulated.

The usefulness of chemicals (molluscacides) is limited by their toxicity for other aquatic animals (copper sulfate), by expense (Niclosamide), or by the particular ecologic setting in which the snails live. Among these conditions are the expanse of bodies of water and the nature of vegetation, sunlight, soil colloids, etc., which reduce the likelihood of reaching effective molluscicide concentrations. Other approaches have included the raising and lowering of water levels behind dams, draining entire swamps, and applying concrete to the floors and walls of drainage ditches. Biological controls are being investigated and include the use of snail predators, introduction of contagious and lethal snail diseases and the development of populations of competitive snails not susceptible to schistosomiasis. All of these approaches are still considered experimental. It is critically important, however, that practical and cost-effective methods be found to control snail populations in areas of developing countries that are being newly opened for human use through dams and irrigation projects, and where schistosomiasis is spreading widely.

Another theoretically possible approach is to attempt to control the numbers of miracidia or cercariae, but these aquatic forms are present for such a short time that any control measures directed at them would require an intensive and continuous application of molluscicides or the use of some form of a slow chemical release mechanism. Efforts are also underway to develop attractants and decoys for these "fleeting forms" of the parasite, but the practicality of such approaches has not yet been demonstrated.

Finally, schistosomes can be attacked in the human host by chemotherapy aimed at schistosomula or the adult stages. Although therapy for individual human cases of schistosomiasis is fairly successful (particularly for early cases), mass chemotherapy is not an effective overall disease control measure. Some of the reasons are: difficulty reaching all persons in a given community, toxicity associated with drug use, need for repeated therapy, and continued re-exposure and reinfection of the population by infested water. Since it is chiefly the eggs which stimulate the destructive host immune response, chemotherapy could theoretically be aimed at sterilizing adult schistosomes (a "pill" for the worm, if you will), and this technique is being investigated. Other possible control measures include production of an enhanced (lethal) human immune response to cercaria penetration or schistosomulum migration, and methods for altering the adult worm's ability to remain effectively "hidden" from the human immune system for long periods of time, allowing for prolonged mating and oviposition.

Both from the clinical and epidemiological viewpoints, total prevention of infection should not be regarded as the major goal of control measures. In most endemic areas, it would be acceptable to begin by attempting to reduce transmission rates and the intensity of schistosomiasis infections.

What method to interrupt the schistosome life cycle would seem to be most practical in the Ugandan village described above where S. mansoni is endemic?

Use of privies for human defecation (if culturally and economically practical), or at least development of the habit of defecation at some distance from the river. Obviously, this approach would require intimate knowledge of socio-cultural habits and beliefs, as the basis for a careful strategy for health education. Selective treatment of persons with heavy worm burdens should also be considered.

Avoidance of human contact with river water is currently impractical, as are the other methods described for chemical control of snail populations. (This particular Ugandan village is not the site for development of a major social or agricultural project). Provision of a safe water supply for domestic purposes should also be considered.

UNDERLYING CONCEPT

There are many experimental approaches to the control of schistosomiasis, but most are currently impractical for the typical village setting in developing countries. See p. 34 for details. The basic methods being attempted are snail control (or eradication), preventing human skin from con-tacting infested water, provision of "safe" water supplies, preventing human (and animal) excreta from contaminating water sources, and selective use of chemotherapy.

If there are portions of the schistosome life cycle which are not clear to you, return to the schistosome diagram on page 31 and review the phases of the life cycle.

A FINAL CHECK

1. In the diagram on the opposite page, points "A" through "F" represent the basic life cycles of schistosomes and points "G" through "K" indicate the resulting human health problems from schistosomiasis. In the space below, please label each point.

A _____

B _____

C _____

D _____

E _____

F _____

G _____

H _____

I _____

J _____

K _____

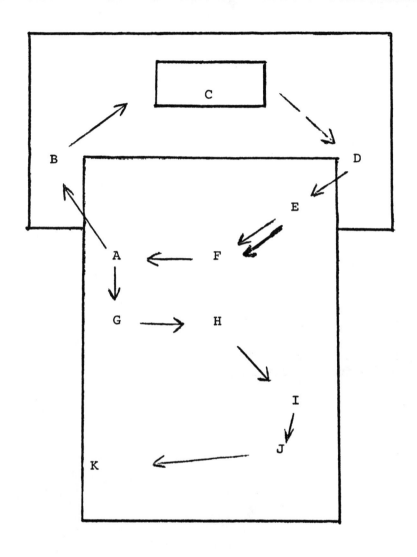

A. Egg
B. Miracidium
C. Sporocyst
D. Cercaria
E. Schistosamula
F. Schistosome pair
G. Eggs in tissue
H. Granulomata, fibrosis
I. Organ damage
J. Irreversibility
K. Death

FINAL NOTE

Please review your response to the question on page 7:
"List the major questions about schistosomiasis which you
would like to have answered by the end of this instructional
unit?" If any of your own specific questions have not been
adequately answered, please note them here and plan to discuss
them with your instructor (you may also wish to consult the
list of suggested further reading).

SUGGESTED FURTHER READING

In addition to standard textbooks of internal medicine, parasitology and infectious diseases, the following are useful references:

Ansari, N. (editor), Epidemiology and Control of Schistosomiasis (Bilharziasis). S. Karger, Basel, 1973.

Gilles, H. M. et al., Results of a 7-year snail control project on the endemicity of S. hematobium infection in Egypt, Ann. Trop. Med. Parasitol., 67: 45-65, 1973.

Hoffman, D. B., Jr. and Warren, K. S., Schistosomiasis IV: Condensations of the Selected Literature 1963-1975, Washington, D. C., Hemisphere, 1977.

Jordan, P. and Webbe, G. Human Schistosomiasis, Charles C. Thomas, Springfield, Illinois, 1969.

Jordan, P., Epidemiology and control of schistosomiasis, Brit. Med. Bull., 28: 55-59, 1972.

Ongom, V. L. and Bradley, D. J., Epidemiology and consequences of S. mansoni infection in West Nile, Uganda. Trans. Roy. Soc. Trop. Med. Hyg., 66: 835-851 and 852-863, 1972.

Stanley, N. F. and Alpers, M. P. (editors), Man-made Lakes and Human Health, Academic Press, London, 1975.

WHO: Measurement of the Public Health Importance of Bilharziasis: Report of a WHO Scientific Group, WHO Tech. Rep. Series, No. 349, Geneva, 1967.

WHO: Schistosomiasis Control: Report of a WHO Expert Committtee. WHO Tech. Rep. Series, No. 515, Geneva, 1975.

UNIT III/5: PARASITIC DISEASES II. OTHERS

BY

MICHAEL M. STEWART, M.D., M.P.H.
RICHARD H. MORROW, JR., M.D.

CONTENTS

(NOTE: Unit III/4 is a prerequisite for this unit. If you have not yet completed Unit III/4, please do so now, before continuing with Unit III/5)

INTRODUCTION

The previous instructional unit provided detailed information on one parasitic disease, schistosomiasis. This unit is more broadly concerned with environmental and behavioral factors which are related to the occurrence of a number of different human parasitic diseases. The concepts and information presented in this unit will be most useful if you have already had some basic exposure to medical parasitology. This unit is not a summary of, or a substitute for, such a basic course, and it is selective rather than comprehensive in scope.

EDUCATIONAL OBJECTIVES

The aim of this unit is generally to present the life cycle of parasites as a form of "biological logic;" that is, to show that most parasitic life cycles are variations on central biologic themes. It is critical that these themes be understood in order to understand the life cycle of a given parasite and to recognize the particular ways in which humans expose themselves to disease. Upon completing the unit you should be able to:

(1)   Diagram the life cycle of a given parasite
(2)   Name the major components in the life cycle for that parasite
(3)   Identify the different points of risk for humans, and
(4)   Recognize types of intervention that can be employed to prevent human disease.

CLASSIFICATION OF PARASITIC DISEASES

Classification is an important technique in medical problem-solving. Much of your time as a physician will be spent classifying patients into the most specific diagnostic categories which the available data will allow. For example, a patient with fever, cough and chest pain might be initially diagnosed (classified) as having a "lower respiratory infection". With more precise data available (personal and epidemiological history, bacteriological studies, X-rays, blood chemistries, serology, skin tests, etc.), such a patient could eventually be diagnosed as having one of perhaps 100 different infectious diseases (or a number of non-infectious diseases).* The importance of arriving at a correct diagnostic classification for a patient with these presenting problems is obvious: appropriate treatment depends on it, as well as prevention of the spread or recurrence of an infection. Thus available data are used to classify a clinical problem in such a way that the most appropriate action can be taken.

Keeping in mind the major subject of this unit (human parasitic diseases), try to name two parasitic diseases (diseases caused by protozoa or helminths) which may present clinically with the symptoms described above, that is, fever, cough and chest pain:

1.

2.

---

*The 1976 epidemic of "Legionnaire's Disease" in Philadelphia is dramatic testimony to the wide range of diagnostic possibilities for a set of presenting symptoms which initially suggest lower respiratory tract infection.

SUGGESTED RESPONSES:

Almost any infecting organism, parasitic or other, can produce fever, and many diverse pathological processes within the thorax can produce cough or chest pain. Human parasites which could involve various thoracic organs or tissues so as to produce this set of symptoms include (among others):

1. _Paragonimus westermani (lung fluke). Adult forms encapsulate within human lung tissue._

2. _Ascaris lumbricoides (intestinal roundworm). Larval forms passing through the pulmonary capillaries break out into the alveolar sacs and pass up through the large airways to the pharynx, eventually being swallowed as part of their life cycle in humans._

3. _Strongyloides stercoralis (intestinal threadworm). Similar to ascaris in that larval forms break out from pulmonary vessels into the lungs and migrate up the airways to the pharynx where they are swallowed._

4. _Entamoeba histolytica (intestinal protozoan). Amebic abscesses of the liver (particularly of the upper part of the right lobe) can extend directly into the pleuropulmonary area, although this is relatively infrequent._

We will return to each of these parasites later in this unit, but here it is important to note that the major "classification question" under consideration so far has been: what human parasites can invade thoracic structures and produce fever, cough and chest pain?

Human parasites, including those mentioned above, can be classified in a number of other useful ways, in addition to the particular tissues which they invade and the clinical symptoms which they produce.

Based on your own medical knowledge to date, list at least three other ways in which pathogenic human parasites could be usefully classified:

1.

2.

3.

Human parasites can be usefully classified in the following ways (among others):

1. *by symptoms of disease produced*
2. *by organs and tissues involved*
3. *by frequency of disease in different population groups*
4. *by geographic location of specific infections*
5. *by degree of involvement of arthropod vectors in transmission to humans*
6. *by degree of involvement of other animal hosts, either as reservoirs of infection or as necessary components in parasitic life cycles*
7. *by means of prevention or control*
8. *by standard binomial biological nomenclature*

The above answers could be regarded as indicating the major spheres of interest of the following specialists:

1. clinicians
2. pathologists
3. epidemiologists
4. medical geographers
5. entomologists
6. malacologists (snail experts), veterinarians, etc.
7. public health specialists
8. biologists

However, any person seriously interested in the ecology of parasitic diseases should be acquainted with certain basic information in these various fields. The importance of human parasitic diseases on a world scale is so great (approximately 25% of the world population is infected with one or more parasites at any given time) that the combined efforts of the above disciplines, as well as others, will be necessary if the impact of these diseases on human communities is to be clearly defined and adequately controlled.

A summary of the standard zoological classification of important human parasites can be found in most textbooks of parasitology and will not be repeated here in detail. In simple outline, the basic unit of zoological classification is the species. Closely related species are grouped into a Genus. These two groupings, Genus followed by species, form the basis of the binomial nomenclature which dates from the time of Linnaeus; e.g. Schistosoma mansoni. Continuing into higher-level groupings, related genera form a family, related families an order, related orders a class, related classes a phylum, and (finally) related phyla form a kingdom. This scheme of hierarchical biological classification basically reflects the notion of a progression from simple to increasingly complex criteria for the ordering of biological organisms. There are many unsettled points concerning the details of such biological classification, and as biological knowledge increases, criteria for classification may change. Nevertheless, this binomial (Linnaean) system of biological classification remains an important method for ordering and indexing a vast amount of biological information.

Human parasitic diseases are caused by protozoa and helminths. The phylum Protozoa is comprised of single-celled organisms including the following which are pathogenic for humans: giardia, trichomonas, leishmania, trypanosoma, ameba, plasmodium, and toxoplasma species. The phylum Platyhelminthes (flatworms) is comprised of multi-celled organisms, bilaterally symmetrical and usually flattened front to back. Flatworms parasitic for man include two classes, Trematoda (trematodes or flukes, such as schistosome, fasciola, paragonimus and clonorchis species), and Cestoidea (cestodes or tapeworms, such as taenia, echinococcus and diphyllobothrium species). The phylum Nematoda (nematodes or roundworms) is comprised of unsegmented, bisymmetrical, cylindrical roundworms. Examples are trichinella, strongyloides, ancylostoma, necator, ascaris and filaria species.

Thus from a practical viewpoint, all human parasites of major
medical importance are members of one of three phyla:

1. Protozoa

2. Roundworms

3. Flatworms
   a. flukes
   b. tapeworms

These three phyla, plus the phylum Arthropoda (arthropods),
together include those members of the animal kingdom which
form the major subject matter of parasitology.

COMPARATIVE LIFE CYCLES OF TREMATODES

Schistosomes have a life cycle involving three phases:
1) sexual mating of adult flukes and production of eggs within the human host (termed the definitive host, because
reproduction within humans is sexual); 2) asexual multiplication within the snail host (termed the intermediate host);
and 3) two non-reproductive motile free-swimming forms found
in water, the miracidium (moving from egg to snail) and the
cerceria (moving from snail to human). The dramatic changes
in schistosome morphology from one phase to another represent

---

*For a fuller discussion of schistosomiasis, consult III/4,
"Parasitic Diseases I. Schistosomiasis"

ighly successful biological adaptations to radically
different environments, and despite the many possibilities
for interrupting this life cycle, schistosomes continue to be
highly successful species from a biological viewpoint.

There are other trematodes (flukes) with life cycles which are
basically similar to that of schistomes, but which differ in
interesting and important ways. Flukes are traditionally
classified according to the organ that is most affected,
i.e., the "lung fluke" (Paragonimus westermani), the "liver
flukes" (Clonorchis sinensis, Fasciola hepatica, Opisthorchis
viverrini), and the "intestinal fluke" (Fasciolopsis buski).
Figures 1-3 (pp. 10, 13, and 15) show certain differences in the
life cycles of these three flukes from the life cycle of
schistosomes.

PARAGONIMUS

As indicated in Figure 1, (p. 10) paragonimus eggs are
discharged by infected humans (either via sputum or, if
swallowed, via feces) into fresh water, giving rise to free-
swimming miracidia which invade particular snail hosts.
After asexual reproduction within a snail, free-living
cercariae are released. In contrast to the schistosome
life cycle, however, these cercariae do not penetrate human
skin, but enter crabs or crayfish (the second intermediate
host), where they encyst in gills, muscles or viscera in
forms know as metacercariae. When humans ingest uncooked or
partially cooked crab or crayfish meat, these metacercariae
pass through the stomach and excyst in the duodenum,
penetrate the intestinal wall, and gradually (over days
or weeks) migrate through the diaphragm or pleural space into
peribronchial areas within the lung. Here the young flukes
mature into adult worms, each encapsulated by fibrous tissue
laid down by the infected human host. In contrast to
schistosomes, paragonimus and other flukes are hermaphroditic,
with each individual adult worm capable of sexual multiplication and egg production. The eggs then gradually work their
way into the lumen of a nearby bronchiole, to be excreted in

FIGURE 1

BASIC LIFE CYCLE OF PARAGONIMUS

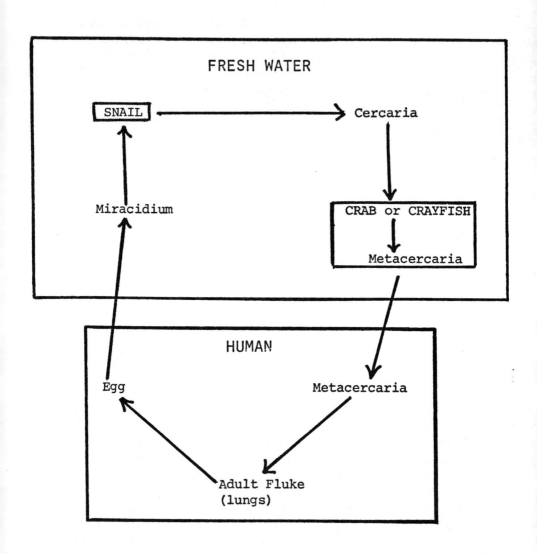

III/5, p. 10

human sputum or feces and to begin the cycle anew.

The major clinical problems caused by lung flukes are those of chronic bronchitis and bronchiectasis, often with production of brownish or bloody sputum. (During the initial phase of migration from the intestine to the lungs, some young forms of paragonimus may also wander to other sites and produce ectopic disease). Definitive diagnosis is made by microscopic demonstration of the characteristic eggs in the sputum or feces. Human paragonimus infections occur in widely distributed endemic foci in the Far East, and to a lesser degree in Central America and Africa. Many carnivorous domestic and wild animals (cats, dogs, rats, wolves, foxes, pigs and others) also commonly serve as natural definitive hosts (and also therefore as reservoir hosts, maintaining paragonimiasis as a prevalent animal infection which can be transmitted to humans whenever circumstances permit).

State four important ways in which the paragonimus life cycle differs from the life cycle of schistosomes:

1.

2.

3.

4.

1. _A second intermediate host is necessary for the completed life cycle of paragonimus._

2. _Humans are infected by ingestion, not by skin contact._

3. _The lung fluke is hermaphroditic, and a single infecting fluke can produce eggs within the human host._

4. _Dissemination of eggs from infected humans can occur via sputum, as well as via feces (but not via urine)._

5. _Unlike S. mansoni and S. hematobium (but similar to the situation for S. japonicum), paragonimus infects an extensive reservoir of animals other than humans._

CLONORCHIS

Figure 2, (p. 13), shows the life cycle of Clonorchis sinensis, one of several liver flukes. Clonorchis, commonly referred to as the "Chinese liver fluke," is found in humans and fish-eating animals in the Chinese mainland, Taiwan, Japan, Korea and Indochina. Imported fish have also been associated with clonorchis infections in other countries such as Singapore and Malaysia. As with paragonimus, humans acquire metacercarial forms of clonorchis by ingestion, but this time by eating various species of small fresh-water fish (raw, soaked in wine or vinegar, or partially cooked) in which metacercariae are encysted in the skin or flesh. These metacercariae also survive pickling, salting and drying. As with paragonimus, the metacercariae of clonorchis excyst in the duodenum, but those of clonorchis remain in the gut lumen and directly enter the human biliary tree through the Ampulla of Vater, often proceeding to proximal biliary branches within the liver. Maturation to adult forms and hemaphroditic reproduction occur within the biliary system, with deposited eggs thus having ready access to the lumen of the human intestinal tract for further dissemination. With heavy worm

FIGURE 2

BASIC LIFE CYCLE OF CLONORCHIS

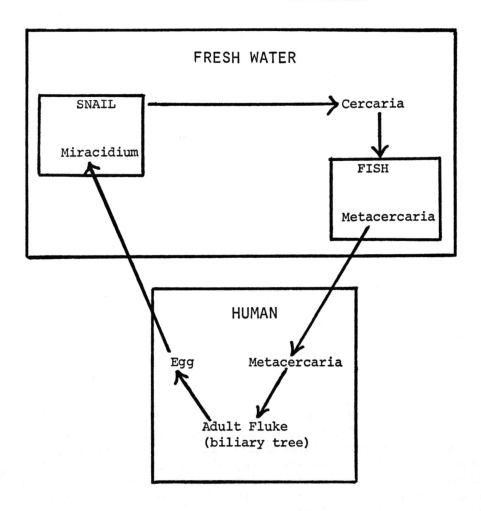

burdens there can be marked liver damage, leading to periportal fibrosis and portal hypertension. Recurrent cholangitis
can result from biliary obstruction caused by adult worms,
and pancreatitis may occur. Clonorchis eggs are discharged
via human feces into the surrounding environment. In contrast
to paragonimus, clonorchis eggs do not produce miracidia until
they have been ingested by an appropriate snail host.
Definitive diagnosis is made by microscopic demonstration of
the characteristic eggs in human feces.

It is of interest to note briefly that infections with another
species of liver fluke, Opisthorchis viverrini, are unusually
prevalent in northeast Thailand and in Laos, and that chronic
infections with this parasite appear to be associated with a
high incidence of primary cancer of the bile ducts
(cholangiocarcinoma) and of the liver (hepatoma). The life
cycle of opisthorchis is essentially the same as that of
clonorchis, with humans acquiring the infection by ingestion
of raw or undercooked fish. In arid northeast Thailand, fish
are a major source of dietary protein, and the prevalence of
opisthorchis infections in many rural villages approaches
100%. It is estimated that altogether some 3-5 million
persons are infected in Thailand, even though this disease is
virtually unknown in other parts of the world.

FASCIOLOPSIS

Figure 3, (p. 15), shows the basic life cycle of Fasciolopsis
buski, the giant intestinal fluke. Fasciolopsis is endemic
in several areas of the Far East. In Thailand, for example,
some 100,000 persons are infected. In this life cycle, discharged eggs release free-swimming miracidia which penetrate
snails, but there is no second intermediate host. Instead,
cercariae released from snails find their way onto the roots,
bulbs, pods or stems of various aquatic plants. Humans acquire
the infection when they use their teeth to crack or peel off
the skins of water chestnuts, water caltrops or other acquatic
vegetation on which these metacercariae have encysted.
Domestic pigs are also an important definitive host. After

FIGURE 3

BASIC LIFE CYCLE OF FASCIOLOPSIS

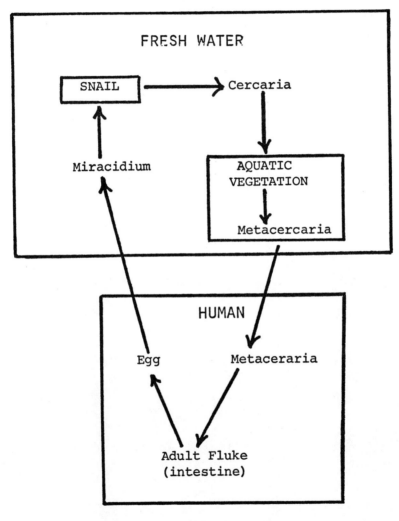

III/5, p. 15

ingestion, metacercariae of fasciolopsis excyst in the duodenum and attach themselves to the intestinal mucosa. Egg
production begins several months later, and eggs are readily
disseminated via the feces. Symptoms are relatively mild
except in extremely heavy infections, consisting mainly of
abdominal discomfort, diarrhea, and occasional malabsorption.
Diagnosis is made by microscopic demonstration of the
characteristic eggs in human feces.

A Quick Review

For each of the flukes lettered A-D in the left hand column below, enter in the blank space the numbers of the appropriate items from the right hand column which pertain to the various trematode life cycles (more than one numbered item may apply to each fluke).

Flukes (trematodes)	Life Cycle Characteristics
A. Schistosomes _____	1. Acquired in humans by ingestion
B. Clonorchis _____	2. Two intermediate hosts
C. Paragonimus _____	3. One intermediate host
D. Fasciolopsis _____	4. Acquired in humans by skin contact
	5. Excysts in duodenum
	6. Miracidium penetrates snail
	7. Snail intermediate host
	8. Direct human-human spread
	9. Free-swimming cercariae
	10. Hermaphroditic adults
	11. Endemic in the U.S.
	12. Eggs passed in feces

SUGGESTED RESPONSES:

A. _Schistosomes_   3,4,6,7,9,12

B. _Clonorchis_   1,2,5,7,9,10,12

C. _Paragonimus_   1,2,5,6,7,9,10,12

D. _Fasciolopsis_   1,3,5,6,7,9,10,12

A Quick Review

For each of the three flukes A-C listed in the left hand column below, enter in the blank space the number of the item from the right hand column which you feel is the <u>single most important step</u> in prevention of human infection:

Fluke

A. Paragonimus _____

B. Fasciolopsis _____

C. Clonorchis _____

Possible Preventive Measures

1. Boil all domestic water

2. Human vaccination

3. Cook fresh water seafood throughly

4. Eradicate snails

5. Avoid eating fish or crabs

6. Sanitary disposal of human excreta

7. Use prophylactic antibiotics

8. Avoid eating raw aquatic plants

9. Avoid direct contact with water

A. *Paragonimus*   _3_

B. *Fasciolopsis*   _8_

C. *Clonorchis*   _3_

UNDERLYING CONCEPT

For all the major pathogenic flukes except schistosomes, humans can be effectively protected by specific changes in common dietary practices.

COMPARATIVE LIFE CYCLES OF INTESTINAL NEMATODES

Nematodes pathogenic for humans fall into one of two general groups: the intestinal nematodes (considered in this section) and the blood and tissue nematodes, the most important of which are the various filarial worms transmitted by arthropods (these blood and tissue nematodes will not be discussed in this unit, however). Most intestinal nematode infections are acquired by ingestion or by larval penetration of human skin, and most do not have an intermediate host. These diseases are generally disseminated by eggs passed in human feces, and are commonly included when "diseases of human filth" are mentioned. Again, in this section, the emphasis is on how humans acquire intestinal nematodes, and on those environmental conditions and human habits which foster these nematode infections.

Figure 4-7, (p. 22, 25, and 29) show basic life cycles for four intestinal nematodes: <u>Ascaris lumbricoides</u>, hookworm, <u>Strongyloides stercoralis</u> and <u>Trichinella spiralis</u>.

As shown in Figure 4 (p.22), humans acquire infective (fully embryonated) ascaris eggs by direct ingestion from contaminated soil. This is common among young children playing in areas around human habitations where indiscriminate defecation has taken place. There is no single activity which increases the risk of ingesting ascaris eggs: any contaminated soil which enters the mouth (by licking the fingers, for example) can cause infection. In those countries where human excreta ("night soil") is still used as fertilizer, the exterior surface of fresh vegetables may be readily contaminated with ascaris eggs. After ingestion, eggs hatch in the human small intestine, and larvae penetrate the intestinal wall to reach small vessels in the portal circulation. Passing through the right heart and into the pulmonary capillary bed, larvae (now only about .02 mm in diameter) break out into the alveolar spaces. From there they pass upward through the airways to the pharynx, are swallowed and return to the small intestine to develop into adults. Here sexual reproduction occurs, and eggs begin to appear in the feces in 2-3 months. Adult ascaris worms are large (15-40 cm. in length) and feed on human intestinal contents. Female worms are prodigous producers of eggs, as many as 200,000 per day. Ascaris eggs can be detected in human feces even if there is only one female worm present. Individual worms are relatively short-lived (12-18 months), so that an infection is self-limiting if repeated reinfection does not occur. Once discharged ascaris eggs reach soil, they require 2-3 weeks of incubation under suitable conditions of warmth, moisture and shade before they become infective for humans.

Clinical pulmonary findings (dyspnea, coughing, ascaris pneumonitis) occasionally occur with a heavy acute infection when large numbers of ascaris larvae pass through the lungs. With light infections, abdominal symptoms caused by adult worms are usually minimal, such as abdominal discomfort or occasional diarrhea. The major clinical problems caused by the large

FIGURE 4

BASIC LIFE CYCLE OF <u>ASCARIS</u>

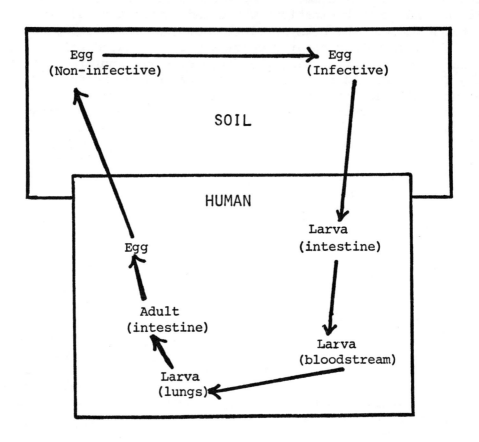

adult worm are 1) intestinal obstruction, volvulus or intussusception caused by a large bolus of tangled worms, and 2) focal damage caused by wandering adult worms, such as bile duct or pancreatic duct obstruction, acute appendicitis diverticulitis, or peritonitis.

Ascaris is a cosmopolitan parasite and causes the world's most common helminth infection (there are numerous endemic areas in the Southeastern United States). It is primarily a disease of children, although persons of all ages can be infected. No intermediate hosts or vectors are involved in the basic life cycle, and because the eggs require a several week incubation period in soil, direct person-to-person transmission does not occur.

A Quick Review

Write in the blank spaces beside ascaris and paragonimus the number(s) of those items listed in the right hand column which apply:

Parasite   Aspects of Life Cycle

Ascaris   _____   1. free swimming larval form

Paragonimus _____   2. acquired by ingestion

                                            3. can produce pulmonary
                                               symptoms

                                            4. penetrates a major food
                                               source

                                            5. reproduces within humans

                                            6. reproduces outside humans

                                            7. eggs infective for humans

- -

HOOKWORM

In contrast to ascaris, hookworm infection is acquired by
active larval penetration of human skin. Figure 5 (p. 25),
shows the basic life cycle of the two common forms of hookworm, Necator americanus and Ancylostoma duodenale (we will
simply use the term hookworm for both, since in most respects
they are similar).

One major difference between the life cycles of hookworm
and ascaris is the existence of a larval form of hookworm in
soil. Following discharge of eggs into favorable soil
conditions (proper moisture, shade, warmth), hookworm eggs
hatch into first-stage (non-infective) larvae which feed on
soil debris and bacteria. In 8-10 days they mature into
second-stage (infective) larvae which no longer feed on their
surrounding environment but await the opportunity to penetrate
human skin. Unless moved by external forces (such as a
passing animal), hookworm larvae remain within a few inches
of the original site of egg deposition. They can remain
viable for several weeks after becoming infective, but are
destroyed by extremes of both dryness and wetness.

Once the larvae have penetrated human skin (usually on or
around the foot), they enter the blood stream and follow
the same route as ascaris to the small intestine. Adult
females begin producing eggs within 1-2 months. Adult forms
attach themselves to the intestinal mucosa and feed on human
blood. The major clinical problem caused by moderate or
heavy hookworm infection is progressive hypochromic,
microcytic iron-deficiency anemia. The degree of anemia is
proportional to the number of adult worms present (or "worm
burden"). This anemia can be treated with supplemental iron,

FIGURE 5

BASIC LIFE CYCLE OF <u>HOOKWORMS</u>

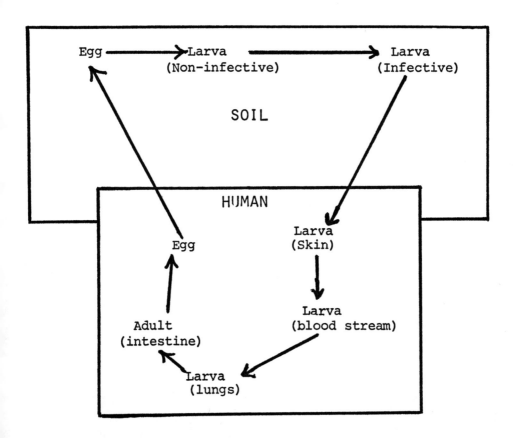

but since hookworms are relatively long-lived (several years), the most effective therapy also involves eliminating the worms from the intestinal lumen (several drugs are effective against hookworms).

Hookworm, like ascaris, is also a cosmopolitan parasite, is also endemic in the southern U.S., and is estimated to infect some 700 million persons around the world.

A Quick Review

Which of the following steps would be rational methods for prevention of hookworm infections?

_____ 1. Always wear shoes

_____ 2. Treat infected persons

_____ 3. Boil domestic water

_____ 4. Take prophylactic iron supplements

_____ 5. Proper disposal of human excreta

1, 2 and 5.

1. _Always wear shoes._ _This is rational, and would certainly help greatly._ _However, hookworm larvae can penetrate skin elsewhere (hands, buttocks), and all shoes do not protect the toes, spaces between toes, or dorsum of the foot. Most important, wearing shoes is not economically feasible nor an accepted custom in many areas of the world._

2. _Treat infected persons._ _Treating infected individuals would reduce the number of eggs discharged into soil. However, reinfections can occur, and many infected persons are relatively asymptomatic._ _Mass treatment campaigns have been relatively successful in many areas, however._

5. _Proper disposal of human excreta._ _As with every disease discussed both in this unit and the previous one, this is potentially the most effective method (and the most complex and difficult)._ _It is especially important for parasites such as ascaris and hookworm, however, since these parasites lack animal reservoirs, and if human dissemination of the disease agent can be controlled, frequency of the disease will be reduced._

Number 3 is irrelevant: hookworm infection is not acquired from drinking water. _Number 4 is not rational: prophylactic medication cannot prevent hookworm larvae from penetrating human skin._

STRONGYLOIDES

Figure 6, (p. 29) shows the life cycle of Strongyloides stercoralis. Two new elements are readily apparent. In contrast to ascaris and hookworm, strongyloides has three different life cycles: a free-living cycle in soil, a cycle involving both soil and the human host, and also a cycle of auto-infection entirely confined to humans. This parasite thus exhibits an unusual degree of variability in its

FIGURE 6

BASIC LIFE CYCLES OF STRONGYLOIDES

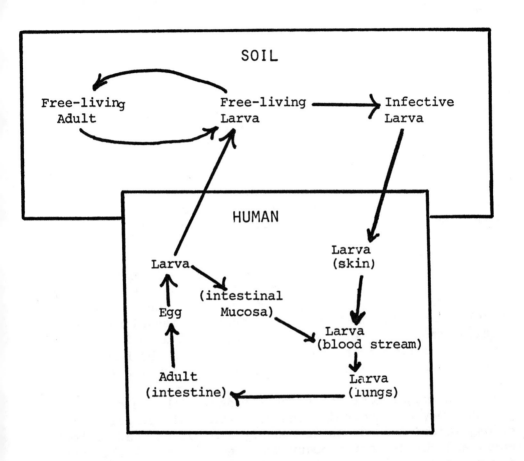

adaptation to different surroundings.

After larval forms are discharged in human feces, they can mature into free-living male and female adult worms which reproduce sexually, eggs being deposited directly into soil. These eggs may again produce actively feeding larval forms which continue the free-living cycle involving no animal hosts at all. Under different environmental conditions, larvae discharged from humans or larvae produced from the eggs of free-living adults can produce larval forms which are no longer free-living but are now infective for man. Infective forms penetrate human skin and migrate to the intestine in a manner similar to hookworm. Male worms survive only briefly before being eliminated in the stool. Fertilized female worms burrow into the mucosa of the small intestine and begin depositing eggs. These eggs hatch in the mucosa, producing larvae which migrate into the intestinal lumen and are passed in the feces, completing the cycle. However, some larvae can mature rapidly to the infective stage while still within the lumen of the distal small bowel or colon. These infective larvae can penetrate the intestinal mucosa or perianal skin without any further phase of development in the soil. They re-enter the blood stream, pass through the lungs to the intestinal tract, and begin a new cycle of invasion, repro- duction, and egg deposition. This cycle of auto-infection thus permits continuing infection in persons who have had no contact with infective larvae in soil for many years.

Man is the major host for strongyloides, although other primates may be involved. The geographic distribution of strongyloides infections is roughly similar to that of hook- worm, and the two often occur together. Tropical climates favor the free-living cycle, while the soil-human-soil cycle is more common in temperate climates. Auto-infection may occur anywhere. Disseminated strongyloidiasis may occur in patients with inapparent or mild infections whose immune defenses become altered by disease or by therapy with immuno- suppressive drugs. Diagnosis of strongyloides is more difficult than with ascaris or hookworm, since eggs are not usually present in feces. Characteristic larvae may be demonstrated in fresh feces or by duodenal aspirate. Eggs may be found in a purged stool.

TRICHINELLA

The final life cycle, that of Trichinella spiralis, is shown in Figure 7 (p. 32). In this case, humans acquire the infection by ingestion of trichinella larvae encysted in the striated muscle of an infected animal, usually pigs, but also wild bears and walruses. (Rat-to-rat cycles also occur, as well as other cycles among wild carnivores and omnivores). The cysts are digested out of infected meat in the human stomach, and larvae excyst in the small bowel, rapidly maturing into sexually reproductive male and female worms. Females begin depositing larvae in mucosal tissue within one week. These larvae enter the blood stream and are widely disseminated throughout the human body. Larvae which enter striated muscle cells increase in size and gradually encapsulate over a period of several weeks. These cysts eventually calcify over 1 or 2 years. Larvae entering other tissues eventually disintegrate, causing local inflammation.

Clinical symptoms are numerous and variable, depending on the stage of infection, the organs and tissues involved, and the number of larval forms invading muscle and other tissues. There are many diagnostic tests, including a skin test, serum antibody levels, and muscle biopsy. (Readers are referred to textbooks of clinical medicine for details of the clinical diagnosis, management and therapy of trichinosis).

The trichinella life cycle differs from that of the previous three intestinal nematodes in several important respects. First, the infected human is a "dead-end" host: humans do not further disseminate the disease. (This is theoretically possible, of course, if infected human flesh were regularly eaten by humans or other carnivores). Second, infected animals are both definitive hosts (supporting stages of the

FIGURE 7

BASIC LIFE CYCLE OF <u>TRICHINELLA</u>

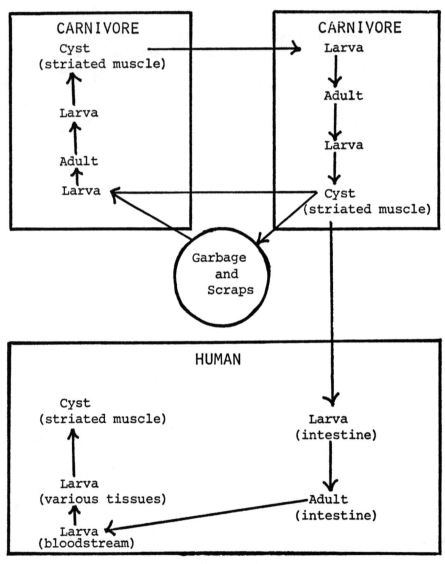

III/5, p. 32

parasite which reproduce sexually) and also intermediate hosts (being required in the life cycle for stages of the parasite which do not reproduce sexually). Third, no free-living form of the parasite exists in soil.

Trichinella-infected domestic pigs are the most frequent source of human infection. The two most important prevention measures, therefore, are to prevent the use of infected, uncooked or undercooked pork scraps as pig food, and to prevent human ingestion of raw or undercooked pork.

There are some other common intestinal nematodes in which human infection is acquired by ingestion of embryonated eggs. These include Enterobius vermicularis (cause of the common pinworm infection) and Trichuris trichiura (or whipworm). Both parasites have relatively simple life cycles: man is the principal host for trichuris and the only host for enterobius; there are no intermediate hosts; neither parasite penetrates beyond the intestinal wall during its basic life cycle; and neither parasite encysts in human tissue. The adult trichuris worms settle in the large bowel, and eggs are passed directly in feces where they can be readily identified. Adult enterobius worms migrate to the perianal area to discharge their eggs. The diagnosis is made not by finding eggs in the stool, but by finding them (with scotch tape) on the perianal skin.

UNDERLYING CONCEPT

Diseases caused by intestinal nematodes, whether acquired by ingestion or by larval penetration of human skin, are closely related to habits of human sanitation.

CESTODES AND PROTOZOA

The three other large groups of human parasites-cestodes (tapeworms), protozoans, and blood and tissue nematodes-are not discussed in this unit. However, the general approach wnich has been followed here is equally relevant to these and other parasites: analysis and comparison of parasitic life cycles, with special attention to those environmental determinants and human habits which place humans at risk for specific parasitic infections, and with identification of possible methods for interrupting the different life cycles.

REVIEW EXERCISE

For the parasites listed in the left hand column below, fill
in the blank spaces under the column headings:

	NO. OF INTER-MEDIATE HOSTS REQUIRED TO CONTINUE LIFE CYCLE?	HOW ACQUIRED BY HUMANS?	DOES PARASITE ENTER HUMAN BLOOD-STREAM? (Yes/No)	DIS-SEMINATED VIA HUMAN FECES? (Yes/No)
Ascaris				
Clonorchis				
Fasciolopsis				
Hookworm				
Paragonimus				
Schistosomes				
Strongyloides				
Trichinella				

III/5, p. 35

SUGGESTED RESPONSES:

	NO. OF INTER-MEDIATE HOSTS REQUIRED?	HOW ACQUIRED?	PARASITE IN BLOOD-STREAM?	SPREADS VIA FECES?
Ascaris	0	ingestion (eggs)	yes	yes
Clonorchis	2	ingestion (fish)	no	yes
Fasciolopsis	1	ingestion (aquatic plants)	no	yes
Hookworm	0	skin penetration (from soil)	yes	yes
Paragonimus	2	ingestion (crabs, crayfish)	yes	yes**
Schistosomes	1	skin penetration (from water)	yes	yes***
Strongyloides	0	skin penetration (from soil); penetration of GI mucosa	yes	yes
Trichinella	2*	ingestion (meat)	yes	yes

*Perpetuation of the trichinella life cycle requires at least two animal hosts, each acting as both definitive and intermediate host.

**Also spreads via sputum.

***Also can spread via urine.

UNIT III/6: VECTOR-BORNE DISEASES

BY

MICHAEL M. STEWART, M.D., M.P.H.
RICHARD H. MORROW, JR., M.D.

CONTENTS

INTRODUCTION

This instructional unit presents the concept of the biological vector, discusses the general spectrum of vector-borne diseases and the global importance of selected diseases, and provides a framework for understanding the major issues involved in the control of malaria. The main focus will be on ecological factors affecting the life cycles of vectors, the interactions of vectors and humans, the biological complexity of those disease agents which undergo important life-form changes as they alternate between different hosts, the effects of vector-borne diseases on human communities, and certain basic principles of vector-borne disease control.

EDUCATIONAL OBJECTIVES

At the completion of this unit, you will be able to

1. Name the organisms causing major vector-borne diseases and also the vectors that transmit them.

2. List the major steps involved in the control of malaria.

VECTORS IN GENERAL

In a general sense, the term <u>vector</u> can be used to describe the conveyor of a disease agent from one place to another. In this broad sense, there are many types of disease vectors, including a mosquito carrying plasmodia which causes malaria, a human hand contaminated with typhoid bacteria, a sewage leak into a drinking water system, and a syringe or needle carrying hepatitis virus.

Conventionally, mechanical vectors (dirty hands, soiled bed linen, contaminated syringes) are termed <u>fomites</u>. The common housefly and the cockroach, though not usually described as fomites, are also frequently incriminated as mechanical

vectors, transporting pathogens externally as adherent
particles from place to place, and sometimes from host to
host.

In more specific medical usage, however, the term <u>vector</u> refers
to a biological vector and is applied when the transmitting
agent also plays a role in the multiplication or development
of the infecting agent. For the remainder of this unit we
will use the term vector in this specific sense, as referring
to a biological vector. Many of the world's most important
diseases are vector-borne. We have already mentioned malaria,
which is transmitted by anopheles mosquitoes.

PREASSESSMENT

Listed below are five important human diseases which are
vector-borne. The pathogens are also listed. Can you
name the vector(s) required for disease transmission in
each case?

Disease	Vector(s)	Pathogen
1. Relapsing fever	_____	B. recurrentis
2. Dengue	_____	arbovirus
3. Epidemic typhus	_____	R. prowazeki
4. Leishmaniasis	_____	L. donovani
5. Onchocerciasis	_____	O. volvulus

Disease	Vector(s)	Pathogen
1. Relapsing fever	*louse, tick*	B. recurrentis
2. Dengue	*mosquito*	arbovirus
3. Epidemic typhus	*louse*	R. prowazeki
4. Leishmaniasis	*sand fly*	L. donovani
5. Onchocerciasis	*black fly*	O. volvulus

Table 1 gives a list of 20 vector-borne diseases, together with the major vectors and pathogens involved. (Note: although most of the major vector-borne diseases are included in Table 1, this list is not intended to be exhaustive or all-inclusive). You are not expected to memorize its contents; rather, you should recognize from the table the variety of pathogens and the major arthropods through which these pathogens are transmitted.

TABLE 1

SOME IMPORTANT VECTOR-BORNE DISEASES

	DISEASE	VECTOR(S)	PATHOGEN(S)
BACTERIA	plague	flea	Y. pestis
	relapsing fever	louse, tick	B. recurrentis, other Borrelia spp.
	tularemia	deer fly, tick	F. tularensis
VIRUSES	dengue	mosquito	arbovirus
	encephalitis (viral)	mosquito	arbovirus
	hemorrhagic fever	mosquito	arbovirus
	yellow fever	mosquito	arbovirus
RICKETTSIAE	epidemic typhus	louse	R. prowazeki
	murine typhus	flea	R. mooseri
	Q fever	tick	C. burnetii
	rickettsialpox	mite	R. akari
	Rocky Mtn spotted fever	tick	R. rickettsiae
	scrub typhus	mite	R. tsutsugamushi
PARASITES	filariasis, Bancroftian	mosquito	W. bancrofti
	filariasis, Malayan	mosquito	B. malayi
	leishmaniasis	sand fly	L. donovani, L. braziliensis, L. tropica
	malaria	mosquito	P. falciparum, P. malariae, P. ovale, P. vivax
	onchocerciasis	black fly	O. volvulus
	trypanosomiasis, African	tsetse fly	T. gambiense, T. rhodesiense
	Chagas' disease (trypanosomiasis, S. American)	triatomid bug	T. cruzi

III/6, p. 5

All biological vectors of human disease are arthropods which feed on human blood. As Table 1 shows, a wide variety of arthropods are involved, particularly mosquitoes, flies, fleas, lice, ticks and mites.

(1) Mosquitoes (which biologically are a species of the Class of Flies) are vectors for the plasmodia causing malaria, and also for the yellow fever virus, dengue virus and many other arboviruses which cause a wide array of clinical diseases, the most serious being the hemorrhagic fevers and various forms of encephalitis. Mosquitoes also transmit the nematodes (roundworms) which cause two major forms of human filariasis (Malayan and Bancroftian filariasis).

(2) Flies of other types are also an important group of vectors. For example, the filarial agent of onchocerciasis ("river blindness") is transmitted by black flies (Simulium spp.); all leishmania are transmitted by sand flies (Phlebotomus spp.); the protozoan agents causing the two forms of African trypanosomiasis are transmitted by tsetse flies (Glossina spp.); deer flies (Chrysops spp.) transmit Francisella tularensis, the bacterial agent of tularemia.

(3) Fleas are involved in the transmission of the agents of plague (Yersinia pestis) and murine typhus (R. mooseri).

(4) Bugs (several species) are vectors of Trypanosoma cruzi, the agent causing Chagas' disease, or South American trypanosomiasis.

(5) Lice transmit the agents of epidemic typhus (R. prowazeki) and relapsing fever (Borrelia recurrentis).

(6) Ticks transmit the rickettsial agents of Rocky Mountain spotted fever (R. rickettsiae) and Q fever (C. burnetti), as well as F. tularensis.

(7) Mites transmit the rickettsial agents of scrub typhus (R. tsutsugamushi) and rickettsialpox (R. akari).

The ecologic factors which determine the geographic distribution and frequency of these many different human diseases are, of course, closely related to the life cycles and habits of the various arthropod vectors involved, as well as to the biologic requirements of the specific disease agents and to the risk of exposure and degree of susceptibility of human population groups. The geographic distribution of each of these human diseases reflects the range of particular ecologic settings which will support continued reproduction of the arthropod vector, the arthropod's acquisition of the infecting agent, and close enough contact between the vector and susceptible humans to maintain continuing disease transmission.

UNDERLYING CONCEPTS

1. *Vector-borne disease agents are not merely "passengers" in the arthropod vector: they multiply and develop within the vector.*

2. *A wide variety of arthropod vectors are essential in the continued transmission of many different agents of human disease.*

DIVERSE NATURE OF ARTHROPODS

Arthropods are the most numerous and diverse phylum in the animal world. If the ultimate measure of biological success is survival, then arthropods are nature's success story. The arthropod vectors listed above in Table 1 are all members of two classes, arachnids (ticks and mites) and insects (lice, bugs, flies and fleas). Other arthropod classes and species also play a role in human illness, including arachnids such as venomous scorpions and spiders, and various crustaceans which serve as intermediate hosts in the life cycles of certain parasites (but <u>not</u> as vectors which actively transmit parasites to humans).*

Arthropods which act as true biological vectors both acquire and transmit the disease agent in the process of feeding on vertebrate blood. It is thought that most vector-borne disease agents initially were parasites of the invertebrate arthropod vector itself followed by gradual involvement of the vertebrates providing the blood meal to the vector. Humans became involved even later in the agent-vector-animal relationship. By now, however, many arthropod vectors have developed intimate relationships with humans, and they seek human blood meals regularly or whenever the opportunity arises, readily acquiring and transmitting certain pathogens in the process.

TICKS AND MITES

Among the class of arachnids, ticks and mites are important vectors of human disease agents, particularly rickettsiae and arboviruses. All members of both families of ticks (the hardbodied and softbodied) feed on blood from vertebrate hosts during their active stages after hatching as larvae. Hardbodied ticks pass through three developmental stages. During each stage they remain attached to one host, engorging themselves with blood, and swelling to many times their fasting size before dropping off to prepare for the next

---

* Examples of this group of crustaceans would be crayfish and crabs, which serve as second intermediate hosts for the development of the lung fluke <u>Paragonimus westermani</u>. The fluke does not multiply in the crustacean, nor does the crustacean seek out man as a food source and transmit the fluke in the process. On the contrary, man ingests the lung fluke after seeking out the crustacean and using it for food. These crustaceans are therefore not true biological vectors of <u>P. westermani</u>. See Unit III/5 for details of the life cycle of <u>P. westermani</u>.

stage. Humans generally serve as hosts to adult ticks.
Softbodied ticks, by contrast, feed intermittently, usually
at night, and hide in or near their host's sleeping place
during the day. It is of particular interest that all tick
and mite-borne diseases are basically diseases of animals,
with humans not playing an essential role in continued
transmission of the infecting agent between the vector and
other vertebrate hosts.

LICE

Among insects, which are the most numerous of the arthropods,
many are vectors of human diseases. Three species of sucking
lice feed on humans, the body louse, head louse, and crab
louse, but only the body louse serves as a biological vector
(for the rickettsial agent of epidemic typhus and the spiro-
chete causing relapsing fever). Lice have a simple life cycle
going from eggs through successive moults to adults, a cycle
requiring 20-30 days.

All stages feed exclusively on blood and all species of lice
are highly host-specific. Body lice live in clothing and
feed on blood once or twice a day. They proliferate under
conditions of poor personal hygiene and overcrowding, particularly in colder climates where heavy clothing is worn.
Typhus has caused devastating epidemics in the past, frequently
during wartime or following disasters such as earthquakes,
floods or famines where overcrowding and poor sanitation
favor proliferation of lice.

Effective means of disease control are now available through
the use of insecticides (for lice) and antibiotics (for
rickettsiae), and continued transmission of typhus is now
found only in a few places (Ethiopia, for example), so that
the risk of epidemics appears minimal. However, body lice
are found throughout the world, and the occurrence of typhus in
certain areas, together with the possible recrudescence of

clinical typhus in infected persons many years after their original infections (Brill-Zinsser disease) and the fact that most of the world's population is not immune to typhus, together make the risk of future typhus epidemics a real possibility in circumstances of severe social disruption.

BUGS

Among the bugs, it is noteworthy that bed-bugs which, like lice, are quite host-specific and live in close relationship with humans, have not been implicated as disease vectors. The only vectors among the true bugs are species of triatomids ("kissing bugs"), which transmit <u>Trypanosoma cruzi</u>, the protozoan causing Chagas' disease (or American trypanosomiasis). Chagas' disease, though geographically limited to South and Central America, is widespread throughout rural areas of Latin America, and is a major cause of heart disease and sudden death due to cardiac arrhythmias.

The various triatomid species are long-lived, and males and females both feed exclusively on vertebrate blood, although their host-specificity is quite variable. <u>T. cruzi</u> infects a wide range of mammals, including humans. Man can become involved in its life cycle in several different ecological settings. Some triatomid species are wholly domestic, living in the crevices of walls, under bed frames or thatched roofs, and feed exclusively on man and domesticated animals. Other species are peridomestic, biting humans as well as other vertebrates, and some species are wholly zoonotic, living in oppossum holes or armadillo dens.

The domestic species of triatomids makes Chagas' disease a major scourge and the most important cause of heart disease in rural South and Central America. However, even if domestic triatomids could be controlled, the existence of various enzootic cycles guarantees the continuing risk of human Chagas' disease in those who intrude into one of the animal-vector-animal cycles.

FLEAS AND FLIES

Fleas are wingless and domestic, and are limited in their effective range of disease transmission. On the other hand, flies include sand flies, black flies, deer flies, horse flies, mango flies and tsetse flies, among others, as well as numerous species of mosquitoes. Flies are important vectors of many human diseases around the world. Flies are well adapted to serve as combinations of incubators and flying syringes. For example, the agent of East African sleeping sickness (Trypansoma rhodesiense), transmitted by the tsetse fly, also infects certain antelope and other game. The transmission cycle goes from fly to antelope to fly; for the most part, the antelope tolerates infection well. The tsetse is a large, fast flying, vicious biter with a wide-ranging appetite. Humans, if bitten by an infected fly, can be readily affected. Tsetse flies live for many months, and once infected, remain so throughout their lives. Other characteristics of this group of vectors are illustrated by the anopheles mosquito, the vector of malaria.

MOSQUITOES

Of the many thousands of mosquito species, some have adapted to fit virtually every geographic locale in which vertebrates can exist. More than 40 species of anopheles mosquitoes can act as vectors for malaria. Only the female mosquito takes a blood meal. Males survive only briefly after emerging and mating, and they live by sucking plant juices. Females also feed on plant juices, but they must have a blood meal in order to produce eggs. After each egg brood has been discharged (one egg at a time, onto the surface of an appropriate water source), the female anopheles must obtain another blood meal before its next brood can develop. Under suitable temperatures, eggs hatch within 24 to 48 hours into larvae. At the water's surface, each active larva matures into the pupa stage. Maturation requires at least 5 to 10 days but varies greatly depending upon the temperature, the particular mosquito species, and other factors. The pupa in turn completes its metamorphosis and with its final moult, the adult mosquito emerges. After emerging, the adult males swarm, attracting and mating with females to complete the mosquito life cycle.

UNDERLYING CONCEPTS

1. *Different vectors live in varying degrees of intimacy with humans, and some important vectors also maintain an extensive domain among other animals.*

2. *Arthropod vectors take repeated blood meals from vertebrate hosts and must survive long enough for the disease agent to multiply and develop between the meal resulting in arthropod infection and the subsequent meal which results in human infection.*

MALARIA AS AN EXAMPLE OF VECTOR-BORNE DISEASE

Malaria is one of mankind's most important disease problems. In the 1960's it became clear that the massive campaign for worldwide eradication of malaria which began in the early 1950's would not be successful. Throughout tropical Africa and in much of Latin America and Southeast Asia, malaria continues relatively unchecked. Indeed in some areas where eradication once appeared imminent, such as Sri Lanka (Ceylon) and Guyana, malaria is again resurgent. The World Health Organization has recently abandoned its commitment to the concept of malaria eradication and is now focusing on effective malaria control as an integral component of basic national health services.

A WORKING EXERCISE

In order to arrive at an effective strategy for malaria
control, it is necessary to know what malaria is, the
causative agent and its life cycle, how it is
transmitted, the pathogenesis of human disease and
its clinical presentations, and the impact of malaria
on human communities. The material in this unit is
intended to provide you with this information.

Because this disease pattern is an important one for
international health enthusiasts, the working
exercise on the next page involves an application of
this information about malaria. We suggest that you
tear out this sheet and work on your exercise as
you read. Later, we will return to this exercise
again.

Tear or cut along broken line

III/6, p. 13

WORKING EXERCISE

In the two columns below, list those factors which
you feel might ENHANCE the possibility of malaria
eradication in a particular geographic area, and
those factors which you feel might OBSTRUCT malaria
eradication.

MALARIA ERADICATION

Factors Enhancing   Factors Obstructing

WHAT IS MALARIA?

Malaria is caused by infection with any of four major plasmodium species (P. falciparum, P. malaria, P. ovale, and P. vivax). Malaria is not a single disease. Each of the four plasmodium species has its own distinctive morphological characteristics, a characteristic clinical disease spectrum, particular antigenic stimuli, an expected theraputic response, and a defined geographic distribution. On a global scale, falciparum malaria and vivax malaria are the most important types. We will focus primarily on infection with Plasmodium falciparum, which produces the most severe clinical symptoms and is the dominant malarial species in geographic areas of the most intense infection (tropical Africa).

P. falciparum infection often does not follow the classical textbook description of clinical malaria, which describes regularly recurrent paroxysms of shaking chills followed by several hours of high fever and headache, culminating in profuse sweating and exhaustion. With P. falciparum, chills, fever, headache, and prostration are common, but regularly recurrent paroxyms are not. Symptoms are often unrelenting, and may include localized complaints such as coughing, abdominal pain with diarrhea, and confusion or stupor. The variety of localized symptoms may obscure the correct diagnosis. The possible diagnosis of falciparum malaria in a non-immune individual should be considered a potential medical emergency whenever it occurs. In a non-malarious area, a physician who considers the diagnosis of malaria is obligated to take a careful epidemiologic history and to perform the necessary diagnostic tests.

In endemic areas, the impact of malaria on the local population cannot be stated with precision. In tropical Africa and in those parts of Southeast Asia where this form of malaria is unusually frequent, malaria is generally considered to be the most serious local infectious disease problem. In these areas it is common for three or four out of every ten live-born infants to die before reaching school age. It is estimated that 25-30% of these childhood deaths are directly due to falciparum malaria, and that malaria plays a contributing role in most other childhood deaths. Thus in these areas, malaria is primarily a disease of young children. By the age of four or five, the survivors of repeated malaria infections have developed substantial (though incomplete) immunity. Malaria thus strikes hardest at the same age that diarrhea, measles, and malnutrition are also taking their heaviest tolls. Most deaths among infants and young children in malarious areas are probably the result of malaria plus a combination of these other factors.

MALARIA LIFE CYCLE AND PATHOGENESIS*

The three major components of the malaria life cycle are the human host, the malarial parasite (one of four <u>Plasmodium</u> species), and the anopheles mosquito vector (See Figure 1). The parasite alternately undergoes sexual reproduction in the mosquito (the <u>definitive host</u>) and asexual multiplication in the infected human (the <u>intermediate host</u>). In man there are two phases of multiplication. After initial invasion, multiplication of the parasites first takes place in liver cells. After first invading hepatic cells, the parasite multiplies rapidly to produce many daughter parasites, called <u>merozoites</u>. In about 10 days the liver cells rupture, releasing merozoites into the general circulation. These merozoites then invade red blood cells and begin the second phase of multiplication.

In each infected red blood cell the parasite goes through another multiplication cycle, again ending with cell rupture and release of merozoites into the general circulation.

---

* Note: This section presents the malaria life-cycle in brief outline only. For more detail, and for important differences between the four <u>Plasmodium</u> species, you may wish to review the subject in a tropical medicine text.

FIGURE 1

BASIC LIFE CYCLE OF MALARIA PARASITES

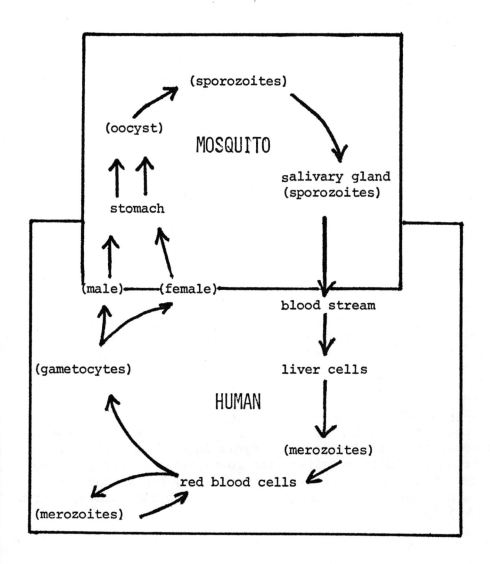

Clinical symptoms are principally related to these repeated cycles of red blood cell rupture and release of merozoites directly into the circulation.

For the parasite itself, there are two biological outcomes of red blood cell invasion by a merozoite. One is the production of more merozoites which invade further human red blood cells and continue to multiply asexually. The other outcome is the production and release into the blood stream of immature sexual forms (gametocytes), the forms of the malarial parasite which are infectious for a mosquito which feeds on human blood.

The factors governing the relative proportions of merozoites and gametocytes which are produced following red blood cell invasion are not well understood, although gametocytes are much fewer in number than merozoites and appear later in the course of human infection. It is important to note that gametocytes must be present in the human circulation in order for biting mosquitoes to acquire the parasite from a human blood meal.

After gametocytes are picked up by a mosquito during a human bite, the male gamete fertilizes the female gamete, which develops into an oocyst in the gut wall of the mosquito. When this oocyst ruptures, the malarial parasites (then in a stage known as sporozoites) disperse within the mosquito and preferentially make their way to the mosquito's salivary glands. Under optimal circumstances this phase of malarial parasite development can take as little as 7 to 10 days, although the actual time depends largely on the environmental temperature. The transmission cycle is completed when an infected anopheles mosquito with sporozoites in its salivary secretions bites a susceptible human host, and introduces these malarial sporozoites into the human blood stream, causing a new infection.

Exercise Review

At this point take a moment to review your working exercise sheet and jot down any additional factors which you think would enhance or obstruct the eradication of malaria. Then compare what you have written with our response on the next page.

Below are some of the factors which can enhance or obstruct the eradication of malaria.

MALARIA ERADICATION

Factors Enhancing	Factors Obstructing
Climate supporting short season of anopheles mosquito multiplication (and shortened life span)	Consistent humid tropical weather providing for continuing anopheles multiplication
Reduction of anopheles mosquito population (by insecticides, etc.)	Resistance of mosquitoes to insecticides
Reduction in human exposure to mosquitoes	Failure of population to avoid exposure to mosquitoes
Widespread use of prophylactic antimalarial drugs	Failure of population to use prophylactic antimalarial drugs
Early diagnosis and treatment of human infections (before development of circulating gametocytes)	Failure of infected patients to seek early treatment for infections.
	Resistance of plasmodia to antimalarial therapy.
	In-migration of humans already infected with malaria into areas with anopheles mosquitoes and susceptible humans.

METHODS OF MALARIA CONTROL

The working exercise should have provided you an opportunity to consider malaria in terms of possibilities for malaria control (as opposed to eradication).

Preassessment

What would you suggest as methods to control malaria?
Name three:

1.

2.

3.

Here are four suggestions that probably include at least some of those you thought of: (1) reduction in human exposure to mosquitoes, (2) human chemotherapy and prophylaxis, (3) human immunization, and (4) vector control. Some further elaboration is in order.

REDUCTION IN HUMAN EXPOSURE TO MOSQUITOES

Reduction in exposure by the use of protective garments, mosquito repellants, and avoidance of malarious areas is commonly recommended for tourists and travellers. However, in endemic malarious areas which offer important sources of local income and livelihood, it is somewhat impractical simply to recommend avoiding exposure. In Thailand, for example, forest and jungle areas where malaria is found are also rich in natural and animal resources (teak, fruits, rubber, various wild animals, etc.). Malaria has been eradicated from the central plains of Thailand, but it persists in the mountainous borders and dense jungle areas where malaria control programs are ineffective and where medical care services are inadequate.

HUMAN CHEMOTHERAPY AND PROPHYLAXIS

There are several antimalarial drugs which are effective in the treatment of clinical malaria. Some drugs are also effective for prophylaxis (prevention). Mass chemoprophylaxis has long been considered as a possible approach to malaria control, but to date this has not been successful on a community-wide basis, principally for logistical reasons. In addition, many experts fear that resistance of plasmodia to available drugs, which has emerged in several geographic areas, may be enhanced by widespread or indiscriminate antimalarial drug use. Other persons are concerned that malaria prophylaxis, without other malaria control measures, may eventually lead to the existence of a large non-immune human population susceptible to a disastrous malaria epidemic whenever other control measures falter.

HUMAN IMMUNIZATION

Another possibility would be the development of an effective anti-malarial vaccine, which, in view of the evidence that substantial protective immunity does develop in infected persons, would appear to be a reasonable possibility. Much active research is being directed to this goal, but nothing that seems promising on a practical level is in sight in the immediate future. One basic problem with vaccine development is the complex antigenic composition of the malarial parasite, which is as yet incompletely understood.

VECTOR CONTROL

Hopes for worldwide eradication of malaria were originally directed in an attack on the mosquito vector, and major efforts have been made to achieve this goal. Until the development of effective chemical insecticides in the 1940's and 1950's, the major means for mosquito control consisted of environmental alteration of breeding sites, such as drainage of swamps and oiling of water surfaces (to prevent early stages of maturation by depriving larvae and pupae of oxygen). These measures continue as important methods for reduction of mosquito populations in some locations, but specific larvicides have now been developed that are much better and much less environmentally damaging than simply pouring oil on mosquitoed waters.

The major purpose of larvicides is to reduce the density of the mosquito population. In places where mosquitoes are inefficient vectors of malaria, reduction in mosquito density may by itself produce a dramatic fall in disease transmission. However, when the mosquito is particularly efficient in malaria transmission (such as with Anopheles gambiae in Africa), even a marked reduction in mosquito density will

have little effect on human malaria. Another factor determining the effect of larvicides in malaria control is the
size of the area to be larvicided and its human population
density. Cost is directly related to the area over which
larvicides are applied, and the per-person cost therefore
varies with the population density in any area. Applying
larvicides to breeding sites in urban areas may be practical,
whereas it would be far too costly for most sparsely populated areas in rural Africa. Larviciding also requires
considerable technical knowledge, and cannot be effectively
delegated to untrained field-level personnel.

DDT, an insecticide dating from the 1940's, was originally
found to be an excellent larvicide: relatively cheap, with
a long duration of activity, and virtually non-toxic to
mammalian species. However, the greatest value of DDT
turned out to be its use as a residual insecticide against
adult mosquitoes. Sprayed onto the interior of houses, it
effectively kills adult female mosquitoes who rest on these
interior surfaces after taking human blood meals.

The important effect of insecticides directed against adult
mosquitoes is to reduce the mosquito life span. Reduction
of average mosquito life span below a critical level will
sharply reduce the malaria transmission rate. The purpose
here is not to eradicate mosquitoes, but rather to prevent
mosquitoes, on the average, from living long enough for
the malarial parasite to complete its developmental phase
in the mosquito before infectious sporozoites appear in the
mosquito's salivary glands. Properly concocted, DDT can be
sprayed onto bedroom walls, ceilings and roofs, and will
act as an effective residual adult insecticide for many months.
The adult female mosquito thus feeds and rest indoors, but
because of DDT does not survive to feed again, and therefore
cannot further transmit malaria.

Malaria control based on the use of DDT as a residual insecticide had the added advantage of making the cost of control proportional to the number of persons or households protected, and, unlike the use of larvicides, the per person cost of spraying with DDT remained constant. Moreover, household DDT sprayers could be rapidly trained and required little technical sophistication or supervision. Finally, spraying DDT on the interior surfaces of human dwellings was far less contaminating to the external environment than widespread use of a chemical on mosquito breeding sites. It was this approach, attacking adult female mosquitoes resting on interior surfaces after a human blood meal, upon which the bold W.H.O. concept of worldwide malaria eradication primarily was based. It was hoped that marked reduction of malaria transmission for a sufficient period (three or four years) would gradually lead to total elimination of the malaria parasite among human populations.

To recapitulate, there are at least three ways to reduce mosquito populations as a strategy for preventing human malaria:

1. Environmental alterations such as draining swamps (where mosquitoes breed) or by other methods of disrupting mosquito breeding sites

2. Applying specific larvicides to breeding sites (to kill young mosquitoes), and

3. Attacking infected adult anopheles mosquitoes through application of residual insecticides to the interior of dwellings and by the wide area use of aerosols.

The value of residual insecticiding for malaria control is evidently dependent upon the post-prandial indoor resting behavior of the female mosquito. There are other characteristics which also can affect the efficiency and effectiveness of an arthropod as a vector, and which might provide opportunities for vector-borne disease control. For example, host preference (animals vs. humans), time and place of biting (day vs. night, indoors vs. outdoors), and mosquito life span and transmission efficiency are all crucial factors in terms of potential disease control efforts.

Several biting habit characteristics contribute to an arthropod's potential as an effective vector. Host preference is critical. Obviously arthropods must bite humans to be vectors of human disease. Some are exclusively human feeders, others may feed principally on animals and only occasionally on humans, while some may be indiscriminate.

Other important behavioral characteristics of an arthropod are the time and place of biting. The most effective malaria vectors tend to be nocturnal and to prefer to feed indoors. Further, most of them also rest indoors after feeding, as mentioned above.

In addition to these behavioral characteristics, the life span of the anopheles mosquito is of critical importance. Since the minimum extrinsic incubation period of the parasite in the mosquito is 7 to 10 days, the mosquito must survive at least that long after its first human blood meal in order to become infectious to another person. In most situations, mosquitoes die off at a steady rate, with a given per cent mortality each day, regardless of age. Average mosquito mortality varies with temperature. However, there are major variations in life span among anopheles species, and each species has a preferred temperature range.

Anopheles gambiae, the major vector of Plasmodium falciparum in tropical Africa, under some conditions has a natural daily survival rate of over 90 per cent, providing a comparatively long life. A. gambiae is such an efficient transmitter of malaria that it has been estimated that 1 mosquito per 20 households can maintain malaria transmission, given the high prevalence of human malaria in much of Africa. Many anopheles females average one blood meal every other day. Once becoming infectious for malaria following the necessary extrinsic incubation period, these mosquitoes continue to be infectious with each subsequent bite. Thus the longer lived a mosquito is, the more efficient a malaria vector it will be. An additional factor determining the effectiveness of a particular mosquito species as a vector is the density of that mosquito species in the area. This density in turn is largely determined by the availability of suitable breeding sites.

UNDERLYING CONCEPTS

1. *Malaria transmission is largely dependent on the effectiveness of the predominant local anopheles mosquito species to serve as a vector. Effectiveness of a particular species depends on its biting habits, its average life span and in some cases its density.*

2. *For residual insecticides such as DDT to be useful, the predominant species must principally feed, and rest after feeding, indoors.*

ERADICATION ABANDONMENT

Once having made a commitment to worldwide malaria eradication, why was the World Health Organization forced to abandon its goal?

First, with the immense biological diversity of anopheles mosquitoes it became evident that some species did not conform in their biting habits to the usual pattern; that is, some species bit outdoors and a few bit during the day. Further, a few species that do feed indoors often fly some distance outdoors for their post-prandial rest. Species with these characteristics are not susceptible to residual insecticides sprayed on the inside walls of dwellings.

Second, major ecological changes were identified as accompanying features of "development." In Guyana, for example, eradication had been virtually achieved when abruptly an epidemic broke out. The problem was that a vector species which had formerly fed principally on horses and bullocks shifted its habits to feed mostly on humans after the mechanization of transportation and agriculture. The underlying reason for the shift in the vector appetite was the gradual replacement of the preferred animal hosts by trucks and tractors.

A much greater problem quantitatively in the use of residual insecticides for control of adult vectors has been emergence of insecticide resistance. Throughout the world species after species has developed resistance, first to DDT and then to other insecticides. Often it has been a matter of a relative resistance, but resistance to a low dose level has progressed in many cases to a total resistance. Frequently, species have become resistant in areas where there was extensive agricultural use of insecticides. Rarely if at all has resistance occurred in response to residual spraying of household interiors alone. Most resistance has occurred as a result of specific enzymatic alterations in the metabolism of the larvicide by the mosquito, but some species have developed a behavioral avoidance of resting on areas sprayed with DDT.

A third problem has been the emergence of malaria parasites resistant to chloroquine. Chloroquine has long been used as a relatively cheap and effective oral drug both for prophylaxis of malaria and for definitive cure of patients developing clinical disease. Resistant falciparum strains first appeared in South America in 1961 and later in Southeast Asia, and the evidence is that these resistant strains have been spreading to new geographic locations. The resistance apparently has occurred independently of the use of chloroquine, but widespread use of chloroquine appears to enhance the spread of resistant strains. Satisfactory treatment of patients infected with the resistant strains poses a major therapeutic challenge.

A fourth major problem involves the varied habits of different human populations. In some places and during some times of the year, many people sleep outdoors. In many areas of the world people live a nomadic way of life and have no permanent housing in which insecticides may be applied. In other places, the usual housing material is not suitable for residual insecticiding.

Perhaps the administrative, logistical, and political factors involved in a campaign to eradicate malaria have constituted the most severe deterrents. In many countries, the basic infrastructure of roads and communications necessary for the organization of a disease control program do not exist. Furthermore, countries in different stages of development have placed different priorities on the eradication effort. A successful malaria campaign would have to be simultaneously coordinated throughout a large geographical area; malaria is no respecter of political boundaries.

Finally, in some areas where malaria is unusually prevalent, the biological efficiency of the vector is so great that eradication efforts are bound to fail, since total eradication of the mosquito population is an impossible goal.

UNDERLYING CONCEPTS

1. *Worldwide malaria eradication has been abandoned as an achievable goal for a variety of reasons including: the development of insecticide resistance, the diversity of anopheline behavior, the emergence of drug resistance in malaria parasites, the varying human ways of life, and organizational difficulties related to administrative, logistical and political problems.*

2. *Abandoning of the commitment of malaria eradication does not mean abandoning control measures. Rather, the complex and diverse nature of the malaria problem requires a varied and individualized approach to control involving the appropriate combination of measures for each particular locale.*

FINAL NOTE

Limitations of space and time do not permit detailed discussion and comparison between malaria control measures and those control measures which might be appropriate for other vector-borne diseases. However, you may wish to consider the following questions for your own further investigation:

1) What are the most common vector-borne diseases in the United States?

2) What agencies are responsible for vector control in the United States? How successful are these efforts?

3) What are the lessons (or implications) of malaria control efforts for the control of other vector-borne diseases, both in the U.S. and other countries?

UNIT III/7. POPULATION I

BY

MICHAEL M. STEWART, M.D., M.P.H.
ALLAN G. ROSENFIELD, M.D.

INTRODUCTION

This is the first of two units dealing with population.
These units should be read in sequence, since the material
in this unit on population dynamics and the effects of
population growth rate on health is an essential prerequisite
for the following unit on family planning services.

The overall goal of these two units is to give you a basic
conceptual framework for understanding population dynamics
and demography, for appreciating the general linkages that
exist between population and health, for identifying specific
types of health problems associated with rapid population
growth, and for comparing the ways in which different
communities and societies are trying to deal with these
problems.

These two units are based on the assumption that there
now exists a "population problem" which is critically important on a global scale, and which therefore should be a
major concern to any serious student of international health.

Preassessment

Before proceeding further, use whatever knowledge you currently have to write below your definition of the "population problem." Be <u>brief</u> and <u>explicit</u>. (Note: you will have an opportunity to revise or expand your definition of the population problem later in the unit.)

SUGGESTED RESPONSES:

There is no single "correct" definition of the population problem. You may have included in your definition some of the following elements (most of which are touched on later during this unit):

1) *The absolute size of the world's current population (about 4 billion), the present world population growth rate (about 2% per year), and the increasingly shorter time it takes for the world population to double (now about 35 years).*

2) *The higher population growth rates in poorer (developing) countries as compared to richer (developed) countries, with the consequence that most of the world's population growth in the near future will occur in societies where material and social resources are already relatively limited in relation to need.*

3) *The implications of large populations and rapid growth in terms of future availability of non-renewable resources (oil, coal, etc.).*

4) *The direct and indirect effects of high fertility on the health status of communities and on particular high-risk individuals (particularly infants and women of child-bearing age).*

5) *Differing national perceptions of (and attitudes toward) the expected impact of large populations and rapid growth on social and economic development.*

6) *The complex range of sociocultural, ethical, economic, political and technological issues, some of them highly controversial, which are involved in the establishment of a "population policy" in any country.*

7) The varying degrees of effectiveness, acceptability and feasibility of current techniques for population control and family planning.

EDUCATIONAL OBJECTIVES

At the completion of this first unit, you will be able to:

1) Define the demographic transition and draw a schematic diagram of this process for both developed and developing countries.

2) List at least three personal health problems which are direct consequences of patterns of high fertility.

3) List at least three community health problems which are indirect consequences of rapid population growth.

POPULATION DYNAMICS - GENERAL CONSIDERATIONS

The annual population growth rate (PGR) for the world as a whole is calculated simply by subtracting the crude death rate (deaths per 1000 mid-year population per year) from the crude birth rate (live births per 1000 mid-year population per year): PGR = BR - DR. Birth rates and death rates are usually reported per 1000 persons, but growth rates are usually given in percent. Therefore:

$$PGR\ (\%) = \frac{BR - DR}{10}$$

For any specific population group, the effect of net migration is also important, and any excess of in-migration over out-migration must be added to the excess of births over deaths to calculate the net population growth for a given time period. For the world as a whole, of course, net migration is zero. However, for certain countries and particularly for urban areas in many developing countries, net migration can play a major role in local population growth.

The expected doubling time of a population can be readily calculated from its current growth rate in a way similar to that used to calculate the total number of dollars accumulating in a savings account with stable compound interest but no additional deposits. For population growth, the "rule of 70" is a quick method for estimating population doubling time: the prevailing annual population growth rate divided into 70 gives the doubling time in years. This relationship is shown in Table 1, and graphically in Figure 1.

TABLE 1

PGR (%)	Estimated Doubling Time (Years)
1.0	70
1.5	47
2.0	35
2.5	28
3.0	23
3.5	20
4.0	17

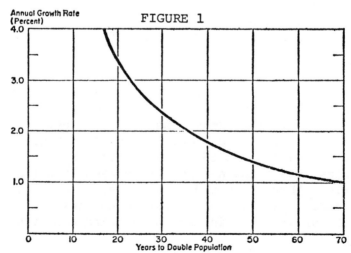

FIGURE 1

Source: The Environmental Fund. 1975. Reprinted with permission.
III/7, p. 6

urrent data for different areas of the world indicate that
here developing countries predominate, population growth
ates are generally in the range of 2% to 3%, whereas in
eveloped countries they are closer to 1%. World population
rowth rate is now estimated to be slightly over 2% (see
able 2).

TABLE 2

AREA	POP. GROWTH RATE (PGR %)	TOTAL POPULATION (BILLIONS)
orld	2.2	4.15
frica	2.8	.42
sia	2.5	2.41
orth America	1.0	.24
atin America	2.9	.33
urope	.8	.47
.S.S.R.	.9	.25
ceania	2.1	.02

ource: The Environmental Fund, 1975. Reprinted with permission.

You should remember that these estimated figures are
aggregates for large geographic regions, and that PGR may
vary widely between different countries. In Asia, for
example, Japan, with a population of some 115 million, is a
developed country with an annual PGR of approximately 1.2%;
India, with a population of some 620 million, has an annual
PGR of approximately 2.0%; and the Philippines, with 44
million persons, is growing at roughly 3% ner year.

The practical and immediate implications of these growth rates for specific countries can be astounding. In India, for example, the total population each day is approximately 35,000 persons larger than it was on the previous day, and well over 12 million additional persons will be added to India's population this year, an increase larger than the total population of Venezuela, or of Hungary. At its current PGR, the population of India will double (to 1.2 billion persons) by early in the 21st century.

UNDERLYING CONCEPTS

India thus illustrates two critical issues in population dynamics: 1) the larger the base population, the greater the absolute increase in total numbers which will result from any given rate of population growth in a given time period, and 2) the higher the growth rate, the shorter the population doubling time, regardless of the absolute size of the population.

From an historical perspective, the world's population grew slowly, at a rate of about 0.0002% per year, until the 17th century. The total world population is estimated to have reached one billion by about 1850. It took only another 75-80 years for the world's population to reach the second billion, with an interval PGR over the previous 150 years of about 0.5%. By 1960, the rate of growth had increased to 1.0% and the population had reached 3 billion. The rate continues to increase and by 1975 the world's population stood at 4 billion. It is expected that there will be over 7 billion persons in the world by the year 2000, assuming that the present PGR of 2.0% per year continues.

FIGURE 2

THE WORLD'S POPULATION GROWTH, PAST AND PROJECTED (ASSUMING CONSTANT FERTILITY LEVELS AS OF 1960-1970).

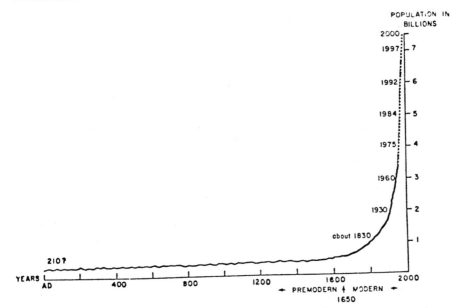

Source: Adapted from The Population Explosion: A Present Danger.

Using the estimated data in the text on the previous page, calculate the expected year by which the world's population of 1975 will reach 8 billion.

Response: 2010 A. D.

8 billion is a doubling of 4 billion. 4 billion is the 1975 world population estimate.

$$\text{Doubling Time} = \frac{70}{PGR} \qquad DT = \frac{70}{2.0} = 35 \text{ years}$$

$$A.D. \ 1975 + 35 = A.D. \ 2010 \ (Answer)$$

These dramatic accelerations in world PGR and in total world population are, of course, major social phenomena, and ones which have different causes and effects in different parts of the world. One important concept is that of the <u>demographic transition</u>. Until the late 18th and early 19th centuries, population size and rate of increase in most societies were regulated by a close and stable relationship between birth rates and death rates. Both rates fluctuated somewhat, with death rates greatly affected by widespread epidemics. However, the two rates remained close in numerical value over long periods, with both rates in the range 35-50/1000, and with barely detectable growth rates.

In the 18th and particularly in the 19th century, however, many of the more developed countries in Europe began to experience a gradual but steady fall in death rates. This decline in mortality preceded major advances in modern medical technology by about 100 years, and appears to have been due largely to factors related to the industrial revolution, particularly improved sanitation and others such as better living conditions, improved housing, better nutrition, and other factors accompanying socioeconomic development. As death rates declined, there was also a subsequent brief period during which birth rates increased slightly.

Can you think of one or two reasons why a fall in the death rate in a given society might contribute to a slight increase in the birth rate during the next generation?

1)

2)

1) *A fall in infant and childhood death rates may enable more female children to survive to the age of child-bearing, thus increasing the pool of potential mothers.*

2) *Increased life expectancy (which is a natural corollary of a decline in a society's crude death rate) increases the probability that women will survive through the entire reproductive period of their lives, and will therefore have the opportunity to bear more children.*

In European countries, after the gradual fall in death rates began, and after the brief period when birth rates appear to have risen slightly, birth rates then began to fall steadily. As shown in Figure 3 (which is a schematic diagram only),

FIGURE 3

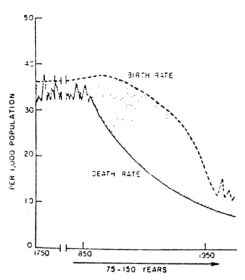

DEVELOPED COUNTRIES

Source: A. R. Omran, Community Medicine in Developing Countries, p. 103. Springer Publishing Co., 1974. Reprinted with permission.

The lag time between the declines in death rates and birth
rates led to a period of several generations of more rapid
population growth. Both rates eventually stabilized at
lower levels, and the annual population growth rate was
sharply reduced. By the present time, crude birth rates
in most countries of Europe and North America are in the range
of 13 - 18/1000 per year and death rates are between
? - 12/1000, with only small annual changes and fairly
stable population growth rates of 1% or less.

The demographic transition, as outlined above, was a several
stage period of adjustment from high levels of both birth
and death rates to significantly lower and stabilized levels.
It should be noted that the steady fall in birth rates which
occurred during the 19th and early 20th centuries also
preceded modern medical technology and the availability
of effective personal health services. There were undoubt-
edly many factors associated with this reduction in
fertility* and the consequent limitation of completed family
size.

List below two factors which you think could have directly
contributed to falling birth rates during the demographic
transition in Europe:

1)

2)

---

*Fertility rate = numbers of live births per year per 1000
women of child-bearing age. It may also be expressed as
age-specific fertility rate (total number of live births
per year per 1000 women of a particular age group) or as
total fertility rate (the sum of age-specific fertility
rates of all women by single years of age, representing
the hypothetical number of births that would occur per 1000
women if they all went through their reproductive lives
with age-specific fertility rates of a given year).

SUGGESTED RESPONSES:

1)   *Delayed marriage (shorter period for child-bearing)*

2)   *Widespread practice of abortion*

3)   *Effective birth control techniques*

4)   *Prevalent infertility (such as from venereal disease, other chronic diseases, anemia, malnutrition, etc.)*

In fact, available evidence indicates that in most countries, birth control was widely practiced well before the availability of the condom, pill, IUD or other popular methods of contraception. The predominant birth control technique was <u>coitus interruptus,</u> or withdrawal. Other than abstinence, couples had little alternative. It is estimated that coitus interruptus, well-practiced, is probably as effective as the condom or the diaphragm. Extra-legal abortion also appears to have been widely practiced, as well as infanticide, in certain societies.

This process of demographic transition is currently proceeding in a different manner in most developing countries. As shown schematically in Figure 4, birth rates and death rates both remained high in many areas well into the 20th century.

FIGURE 4

LESS DEVELOPED COUNTRIES

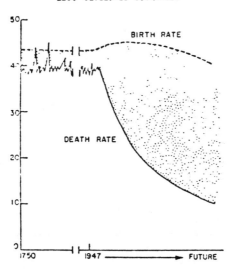

Source: A.R. Omran in Community Medicine in Developing Countries, p. 103. Springer Publishing Company, 1974. Reprinted with permission.

Following World War II, however, death rates began to fall dramatically, largely as a result of aggressive public health campaigns against controllable diseases such as malaria, smallpox and cholera, as well as rapid improvements in nutrition, environmental and food sanitation, and the availability of personal health services including immunizations, antibiotics, and adequate hospital facilities.

However, the demographic transition in these countries is obviously incomplete. Death rates have fallen far and fast, but birth rates have only recently begun to move consistently downward. During this lag period, these countries are experiencing an inevitable surge of rapid population growth which will not abate until well after birth rates have declined to levels low enough so that the difference between birth rates and death rates is small (10/1000 or less). Because of the rapidity and magnitude of the fall in death rates which has already taken place, it is clear that total population growth in developing countries at this stage of the demographic transition will be determined primarily by the extent of future reductions in birth rates. This is why population control and limitation of family size are so important on an international scale.

A SPECIFIC EXAMPLE-THAILAND

Now consider the situation of one particular country where the population problem can be described and discussed in more specific terms.

<u>Name</u>: Thailand
<u>Location</u>: Southeast Asia, surrounded by Burma, Laos, Cambodia, and Malaysia, with extensive coastlines on the Gulf of Siam and the Indian Ocean.
<u>Age</u>: Approximately 800 years
<u>Size</u>: Population 43 million, area 200,000 sq. mi.*
<u>Chief Complaint</u>: Population increasing too rapidly
<u>Present Illness</u>: For most of this nation's existence, the rate of population increase has been very gradual. From its national birth some 800 years ago (the exact date is not known with certainty) it took until 1910, the date of the first national population census, to reach a total population of 8 million people. By that time signs of rapid population growth were already apparent, although symptoms were minimal.

---

*Compare Texas, 270,000 sq. mi., population of 12.2 million; and California, 160,000 sq. mi., population of 21.2 million.

During the next 32 years, the population doubled, reaching 16 million in 1942. Another 8 million people were added by 1957, and another 8 million by 1966. As of 1976, well over one million people are being added to the population each year, and the total national population is now approximately 43 million. Projections based on the present rate of growth predict a population of 70-80 million people by the year 2000. (It is likely that none of these census figures or population estimates are very precise, although their accuracy has probably been improving in recent decades).

Based on the material already provided to you in this unit, identify three major factors which may be contributing to rapid population growth in Thailand. Also, see if you can identify some of the likely health-related consequences of rapid population growth.

Contributing Factors	Possible Health-Related Consequences
1)	1)
2)	2)
3)	3)

Contributing Factors	*Possible Health-Related Consequences*
1) *recent rapid fall in death rate (with greater probability of childhood survival and increased life expectancy)*	1) *increased need for health services*
2) *continued high birth rate*	2) *health problems accompanying rapid urbanization*
3) *more complete recent census data*	3) *increase in abortions (and their complications)*
4) *net in-migration*	4) *increased maternal and child morbidity and mortality*

Note: the health-related consequences in the right-hand column are discussed in later sections of this unit, although most of them are self-evident. Among the "contributing factors" listed above, net in-migration is not a major factor in Thailand's population growth, although substantial migration does occur back and forth across Thailand's largely remote borders.

SYSTEMS REVIEW (THAILAND)

General: This nation has many complaints regarding its general social system, several of them related to the presenting problem of rapid population growth.

Economic Status: Although there are many handsome buildings and flourishing businesses in the capital city (Bangkok), the effects of urban modernization and industrialization are not felt in most of the rural areas where the majority of the population (80-85%) live and work. Average annual per capita income is well under U.S. $200. Families in rural areas (average family size 7 or 8 persons) commonly spend

J.S. $8.00 per person on health care services (4-8% of cash
income), although the government's expenditure on health is
less than $2.00 per person per year.

Education: Less than 20% of the total population has more
than four years of elementary schooling, and functional
illiteracy (cannot read or understand a newspaper) is estimated
at greater than 50%. Although more schools are being built
and many teachers trained, there are far too few places in
elementary schools for all children. Similarly, despite
efforts to increase opportunities for secondary and

FIGURE 5

NUMBER OF STUDENTS IN SCHOOL, BY GRADE AND BY SEX

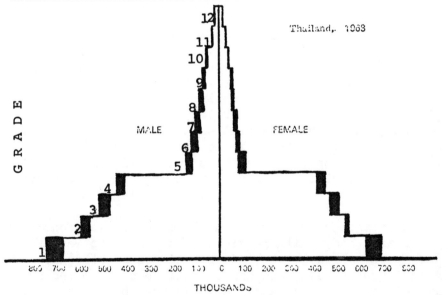

university-level education, the percentage of elementary
school graduates who eventually enter universities is
minute (less than 1%).

III/7, p. 19

Agriculture: Export of rice has long been a major source of
foreign income, and rice-farming remains the predominant
national livelihood. Lately, however, more rice is needed
for the domestic market, with prices much lower than on the
world market. Much rice production is by tenant farmers.
Other important crops include coffee, sugar, corn, rubber
and certain fruits, many of these raised on large estates
with absentee landlords. Agriculture is the economic and
social backbone of the country, with livestock breeding
(pigs, cattle, sheep) of growing importance. However, there
is growing social unrest in rural agricultural areas. One
important problem is that families have increasing difficulty
subdividing family-owned land among living sons. Many young
people are now leaving their rural homes and moving to urban
areas (often into slums) to look for manual or unskilled work
with immediate cash benefits, however low the wages may be.

Social Welfare: Most social welfare efforts are concentrated
in Bangkok (4 million people and growing at a rate of 7-8%
per year) and in a few other outlying urban areas, although
as of 1975 there was no other city larger than 100,000
persons. The urban and periurban slum population of Bangkok
needs these social services desperately, but it is dramatically underserved. Medical social workers, for example, are
virtually non-existent. There is no general provision for
old-age income pensions, nor is there any consistent effort
to provide food supplements to all who need them, to improve
job opportunities or to assist in income supplementation.

Health Care: Although death rates have decreased substantially
in recent years, they still remain high compared to western
countries, particularly among infants and young children.
The national crude death rate has recently been reported as
approximately 10/1000 year and the infant death rate as
approximately 32/1000 (although more realistic estimates for
the infant death rate put it closer to 80/1000). There are
relatively few fully-trained physicians in the country (less
than 6000 in all), and they are largely concentrated in
Bangkok and provincial capitals. Physician-to-population

ratios in outlying and rural areas are frequently as low as 1:50,000 or 1:100,000. In general, modern health care facilities in these outlying areas are seriously inadequate, usually consisting of one provincial hospital and several satellite health centers, each designed to serve a population of some 50,000 persons. Most women continue to deliver babies at home with the help of relatives or "granny midwives" (indigenous, non-governmental and usually untrained). Many mothers die during childbirth, and the maternal mortality rate is unofficially estimated to be 3 to 5 per 1000 live births (10 to 30 times higher than in most western countries).* Large numbers of children die before age 5, and the chances of surviving from birth to age 5 are only about 80%. Some specific high frequency health problems include: 1) diarrheal and respiratory diseases in children; 2) malnutrition; 3) malaria; 4) amebiasis, hookworm, and other intestinal parasites; 5) tuberculosis; 6) trauma and accidents.

SUMMARY

The types of information already mentioned in this unit which are important in characterizing the "population problem" as it now exists in Thailand include, among others: annual population growth rate, crude birth and death rates, population size/distribution, patterns of internal migration, average family size, infant death rate, maternal death rate, frequency of home deliveries. Jot down 2 or 3 other types of information useful in providing a more comprehensive picture of the current population problem in Thailand:

1.

2.

3.

---

*U.S. maternal mortality in 1974 was 14.6/100,000 overall, 10.0/100,000 for white females and 35.1/100,000 for all others.

You could have included some of these in your response:

1) *attitudes toward (and practice of) birth control and family limitation*

2) *Thailand's "population policy"*

3) *availability of family planning services*

4) *abortion practices*

5) *weaning practices*

6) *availability of maternal and infant care*

7) *disease-specific morbidity and mortality data for mothers and young children*

Note: these responses are <u>not</u> intended to be exhaustive. Also, many of these items will be discussed in Unit III/8 on family planning services.

PHYSICAL EXAMINATION   (THAILAND)

General: A reasonably healthy-looking country with wide variations in geography, climate and population density, and major differences between urban and rural areas.

Urban Areas: Many fancy new buildings, but careful inspection reveals that they are often poorly constructed, and many are surrounded by extensive slums, with problems of community sanitation, availability of health services, basic education, job opportunities, etc. Traffic is dense and sometimes impassible. Foreign tourists may be numerous, depending on the political situation.

Rural Areas: Little evidence of modernization is apparent. Most families work a family plot, growing rice and doing other chores by hand. Water buffaloes are a major beast of burden. There is a strong tradition of social stability and community integrity, with a Buddhist temple often forming the center of village activity. "Modern" social services (health, education, agricultural cooperatives, participation in the voting process) tend to play a relatively minor role. There is an active "indigenous" (unofficial, nongovernmentally sponsored) health and medical care system, consisting of spirit doctors, herbalists, granny midwives, and a variety of medical entrepeneurs. Utilization of modern health services is largely regulated by their geographic availability. In many areas, the closest general/family MD practitioner is half a day's journey away.

The People: Signs of mild to moderate malnutrition are generally evident, and kwashiorkor and marasmus (forms of severe malnutrition) can be observed in children in some areas. Many families have at least one child who has died before reaching age five, and interpretation of the reason(s) for childhood death are highly variable. Also, there are many families which have experienced maternal death during pregnancy or delivery, most commonly among primagravidas (women with first pregnancies) or older women with many previous deliveries. Children under age 15 comprise over 45% of the total population, giving a childhood dependency ratio of 90/100. That is, there are approximately 90 dependent children (under age 15) for every 100 working age adults*.

---

*Compare Sweden, for example, where only 25% of the population is under age 15, and the childhood dependency ratio is 32/100.

GENERAL IMPRESSIONS OF THAILAND'S POPULATION PROBLEM

1) Unequivocally high population growth rate, due primarily to a large excess of births over deaths throughout the country.

2) Multiple social problems related to a rapidly growing population, a high childhood dependency ratio, and the phenomenon of rapid and unplanned urban growth in Bangkok.

PLAN

1) Further analysis is required of the specific impact of rapid population growth on the health status of mothers and children (discussed in the remainder of this unit).

2) Major efforts toward fertility control and population stabilization are indicated for social and medical reasons (these efforts are discussed in Unit III/8. Population II: Family Planning Services).

IMPACT OF POPULATION ON HEALTH

The material presented so far in this unit has dealt primarily with the general social consequences of rapid population growth. As countries such as Thailand and India continue to grow rapidly in total population, socioeconomic development (as measured by GNP, for example) is continually diluted by the growing numbers of persons consuming national resources in all sectors (i.e., per capita GNP fails to improve significantly). This check on development is true in the health sector as well. In Thailand, the annual increment in the number of physicians who complete their training and remain in the country to practice is between 200 - 300 per year, or roughly a 5% increase in the total number of physicians. In the face of an annual PGR of 3%, this represents very slow progress in meeting a pressing need for more physicians for a seriously underserved society.

ome of the serious health-related problems of rapid
urbanization have already been mentioned. It is not surprising that urban slums, with inadequate provisions
for human waste disposal, limited supplies of safe water,
poorly constructed dwellings, rapid dissemination of certain
communicable diseases, breeding sites for mosquitoes and
other vectors, and prevalent conditions of family and
community crowding, act as major health hazards to their
inhabitants. In fact, rapid and relatively uncontrolled
urbanization is one of the predominant health problems in
developing countries around the world.

However, there is another aspect of population growth which
must also be appreciated, even though it can be discussed
here only briefly. This is the direct impact of large
families on maternal and child health. Evidence from many
settings indicates that:

1) maternal morbidity and mortality are directly related
   both to maternal age at delivery and to parity (the
   total number of children born).

2) infant (under 1 year) and childhood (years 1-4) morbidity
   and mortality are directly related to the total number
   of children per family, the time interval between births
   of successive children, and a child's rank in the family
   birth order (i.e., whether a child is born early or late
   among siblings).

These associations appear to be relatively constant in
different geographic settings and in families of different
socioeconomic classes.

MATERNAL MORTALITY

Data from Thailand and other countries show that the risk
of maternal death follows an assymetrical U-shaped curve
both for maternal age and parity (maternal death may be due
to such obstetrical complications as toxemia, dystocia,

various types of hemorrhage, or uterine rupture). As shown in Figure 6, maternal mortality is relatively high for women under age 20, falls for women in the age group 20-34, and then rises significantly and successively for women aged 35 and over. Similarly, for women bearing their first child,

FIGURE 6

MATERNAL MORTALITY BY AGE

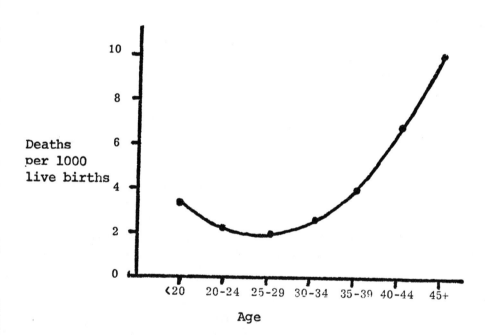

the risk of maternal death is relatively high (Figure 7), falls
for the next two or three pregnancies, and rises rapidly for
all pregnancies after the fourth. The combined impact of these
two sets of data is that maternity presents the greatest risk

FIGURE 7

MATERNAL MORTALITY BY PARITY

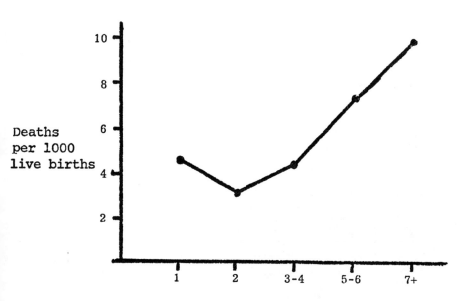

for two particular groups: young women having a first child, and for women over 35 who have already had four or more previous children. It is noteworthy that in countries such as Thailand, where completed family size is large (see Figure 8), some 20-25% of all children are born to women aged 35 and over, and 40-50% of all births occur in women who have already had four or more previous children.

FIGURE 8

AVERAGE NUMBER OF CHILDREN EVER BORN

PER WOMAN COMPLETING THE CHILD-BEARING AGE (1969)

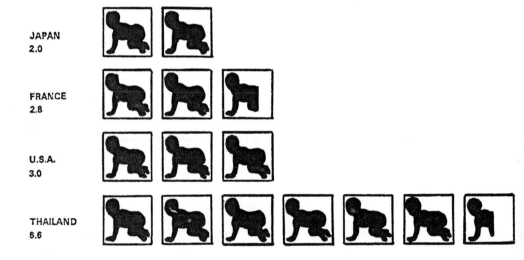

JAPAN
2.0

FRANCE
2.8

U.S.A.
3.0

THAILAND
6.6

CHILDREN AT RISK

Children in large families are also at particular risk.
As already noted, the variables here may include total number
of children per family, the birth interval between successive
children, and the child birth order. In families with larger
numbers of children, diseases such as gastroenteritis and
malnutrition occur more frequently within the family. Physical
and mental development in children are negatively correlated
with the total number of children in a family, as indicated
by such measurements as gain in height, I.Q. tests and age
of menarche. Short birth intervals may lead to early weaning
and increased risk of malnutrition in the child displaced pre-
maturely from the breast, as well as to a "maternal depletion
syndrome" in the mother (iron deficiency anemia, malnutrition,
avitaminosis), resulting from the cumulative and continuous
physiologic stress of pregnancy and lactation which accompanies
short birth intervals. Moreover, infant and childhood mortality rates generally rise with increasing maternal age and
parity and with later rank in the birth order. Thus in
developing countries, where a total of 6-8 children per
family is often the norm, all children in large families are
placed at increased risk of retarded development, illness,
and early death.

The adverse effects of many pregnancies and large families
on children and on women of child-bearing age (who together
comprise some 60% of the total population in many countries)
suggest that birth control campaigns directed at women over
30 with three or more children already born might actually
be viewed (in a manner similar to malaria control or smallpox
eradication) as cost-beneficial solely in terms of
potential reductions in morbidity and mortality rates for
mothers and children. This is not the usual rationale

for family planning programs, of course, but as indicated above, the interrelations of maternal age, parity, family size, birth interval and birth order have many of the features of an "epidemic" which puts certain individuals at unusually high risk.

CONCLUSION

This unit has been primarily concerned with rapid population growth and large family size as adverse influences on the health of communities, families, and individuals. These various factors are outlined schematically in Figure 8.

FIGURE 8

OUTLINE OF EFFECTS OF POPULATION ON HEALTH

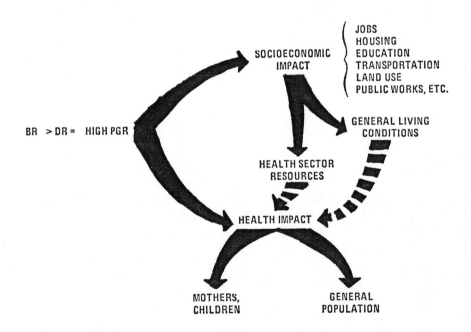

Now list three personal health problems and three community
health problems which are related to rapid population growth
and high birth rates in developing countries such as Thailand:

PERSONAL HEALTH PROBLEMS   COMMUNITY HEALTH PROBLEMS

1)   1)

2)   2)

3)   3)

SUGGESTED RESPONSES:

The following problems are suggested. This is not meant to be an exhaustive list. You perhaps included some not given here.

PERSONAL HEALTH PROBLEMS

1) obstetrical complications (various)

2) maternal depletion syndrome

3) malnutrition

4) retarded mental and/or physical development

COMMUNITY HEALTH PROBLEMS

1) inadequate health care resources to meet growing needs

2) crowding

3) poor sanitation

4) limited education, illiteracy

Finally, please review your response to the Preassessment on page 3 in which you wrote your preliminary definition of the "population problem." You may wish to use the space below to write down (for your own use) any revisions which you feel will improve your original definition.

Revised definition of the "population problem:"

SUGGESTED FURTHER READING

A.R. Omran, "The World Population Problem," in Community Medicine in Developing Countries, Springer Publishing Co., 1974.

J.D. Wray: Population Pressure on Families: Family Size and Child Spacing. Reports on Population/Family Planning, No. 9, August 1971.

Scientific American, September 1974 (issue on "The Human Population"), especially A.J. Coale, "The History of the Human Population."

UNIT III/8. POPULATION II: FAMILY PLANNING SERVICES

BY

MICHAEL M. STEWART, M.D., M.P.H.
ALLAN G. ROSENFIELD, M.D.

CONTENTS

(Note III/7 - Population I is a prerequisite for this unit.
If you have not already completed Unit III/7, please do so
now, before starting Unit III/8.)

INTRODUCTION

This unit on family planning programs (FPP's) could logically
have been included in Category V ("Systems of Health Care"),
but it seemed more useful to place it immediately after
Unit III/7, which deals with the "population problem," so
that a discussion of different approaches to fertility
control could be considered at the same time. This unit
summarizes the major methods of fertility control, certain
aspects of the various approaches used to deliver family
planning services to large population groups, and some of
the complex relationships which exist between availability
and acceptance of family planning services and their impact
on fertility and population growth.

It must be emphasized that this is only an introduction to a
continually changing area of international health. The data
in many cases are rather soft and incomplete, and there exists
a considerable amount of uncertainty about causal relationships between use of FPP's on the one hand, and observed
changes in birth rates and population growth rates in
different countries. There are a number of important
technical issues and controversies in this field which you
may wish to explore further on your own, as well as some
broader economic, social and ethical issues which are beyond
the scope of this unit.*

The basic concepts on which most FPP's have been organized
are straightforward: where high birth rates are associated
with rapid population growth and with high infant and maternal

---

*See P. Reining and L. Tinker (editors): <u>Population:
Dynamics, Ethics and Policy</u>, AAAS, 1975; recent volumes of
<u>Studies in Family Planning</u> (monthly pulication of the
Population Council); and the list of suggested further
reading at the end of the unit.

ortality rates, large-scale delivery of family planning
ervices (1) is socially desirable and (2) will help to
ower birth rates, fertility rates, and population growth
ates, as well as leading to reductions in morbidity and
ortality among mothers and young children.

EDUCATIONAL OBJECTIVES

t the completion of this unit, you will be able to:

) Outline, in schematic form, the major elements in a
   national family planning program.

) List at least three factors which promote, and three
   factors which inhibit, the effectiveness of family
   planning efforts.

) List at least three measures of performance which could
   be used to assess a given family planning program.

) Describe the major characteristics of the five most
   common contraceptive methods used in national FPP's.

HISTORICAL ASPECTS OF FAMILY PLANNING

The modern birth control and family planning movement
n the United States originated in the early 1900's, in
conjunction with a more broadly focused radical movement
which aimed to liberate women and to promote the social and
economic welfare of the working class. Margaret Sanger was
this movement's leading proponent and spokesperson for birth
control. Almost single-handedly she carried the movement for
forward and through her doggedness and determination enlisted
the support of various organized groups, even spending
time in jail as a result of her battle for the social and
biologic rights of women.*

*See Kennedy, D.M.: Birth Control in America: The Career of
Margaret Sanger, Yale University Press, 1970.

Similar efforts began on other continents, led by such persons as Maria Stopes (Great Britain) and Lady Rama Rau (India). Birth control clinics were opened in urban areas, and gradually these services were made more widely available to other women. The post-WWII era then brought with it rapid declines in infant mortality, increased life-spans, and dramatic accelerations in population growth rates, adding a new dimension of demographic urgency to organized birth control efforts. This development, accompanied by the many technologic advances in health care during the 1950's and 1960's, has thus built on the legacy of the earlier "woman's rights" movement to shape the vigorous worldwide family planning and population control movement as it exists today. It is important to note that well organized and officially supported family planning programs in most countries have occurred primarily during the past 10-15 years. For example, even in the United States, specific Federal support for family planning efforts did not begin until 1967, and many court decisions regarding women's rights to contraception and abortion are even more recent.

CONTRACEPTIVE METHODS

From a technical viewpoint, the ideal contraceptive method would be medically safe and free of side effects, 100% effective in preventing unwanted pregnancy, would sustain its effect for as long as necessary, and would be reversible if an intentional pregnancy were desired. From the viewpoint of the individual user, however, the actual acceptability and use of a contraceptive method is likely to be determined by a different set of criteria, including factors such as: out-of-pocket cost; availability and convenience; simplicity and needed frequency of use; degree of interference with sexual activity, libido and life style; specific side effects; conformance with religious beliefs, local customs and superstitions; and mutual acceptance by one's sexual partner. There is not yet any "ideal" contraceptive which meets all the above technical standards and personal criteria for use.

For simplicity, contraceptive methods can be divided into two general groups, traditional and modern methods:

Traditional Methods (not requiring medical intervention)

> abstinence
> coitus interruptus (withdrawal)
> post-coital douche
> prolonged breast-feeding (after prior pregnancy)
> rhythm (safe period)

Modern Methods (chemical, mechanical, surgical)

> condom
> diaphragm
> induced abortion
> injectable contraceptive (depot methoxyprogesterone acetate, or DMPA)
> intra-uterine device (IUD)
> local spermicide (cream, foam, jelly)
> oral contraceptive (pill)
> sterilization (female and male)

In organized family planning programs, greatest use has been made of those methods with the lowest failure rates. The failure rate of a contraceptive method is commonly expressed as follows:

> failure rate = no. of pregnancies/100 woman-years of use

Given this definition of contraceptive failure rate, the "success rate" of a contraceptive method, which can be logically expressed as (1 - the failure rate), is the number of women successfully protected from pregnancy per 100 woman-years of contraceptive use. This success rate reflects several things: the availability of a particular contraceptive method; the degree to which women are motivated to accept it; and their willingness and ability to continue its use once they have started. Since the desired end result

III/8, p. 5

of contraception is fertility regulation, in terms of both
number and spacing of live births, the use of failure-rates
as a final measure of contraceptive effectiveness makes
sense. However, there are a number of other ways to measure
the performance of FPP's, depending on which aspect of a
program is under specific consideration (see below).

Most governmentally sponsored FPP's have relied on various
combinations of the pill, IUD, condom, sterilization, and
abortion. Each of the other methods listed above has major
limitations or disadvantages. Diaphragms are highly
effective if used properly, but they must be individually
fitted initially and then manually inserted before each
sexual exposure. They are also relatively expensive.
Spermicides can be somewhat messy but, again, if used properly can be reasonably effective. Injectable steroid
contraceptives have been used with reportedly great success
in a number of field programs, and have the particular advantages of long action (3-6 months) and in most cases, reversi-
bility after they are discontinued. However, for practical
purposes, they are best regarded as still being in the field-
test stage, since only one or two countries have incorporated
them as a regular feature in a national family planning
program.*

The remaining five methods--condom, pill, IUD, sterilization
and induced abortion--are the most important methods from a
public health viewpoint. Condoms are readily available
commercially, are cheap, and do not require prescriptions
or any sort of medical supervison. Their main disadvantages
are that they are coitus-dependent (i.e., must be used
regularly during every sexual exposure), that they may be
personally unacceptable, and that they have a failure rate,
even when regularly used, of 5-10 pregnancies per 100 woman-
years. In addition, use of condoms requires specific

---

*See Rosenfield A.R.: Injectable long-acting progestogen
contraception: A neglected modality. Amer J Obstet Gyn
120:537-548, 1974.

continued cooperation by the male partner, a factor which does not apply to the other four major methods. One unique fringe benefit of condom use for fertility control is protection against venereal disease, but this may actually serve as a disincentive to condom use as a form of marital birth control, since condoms are associated in some people's minds with illicit sex, prostitution and "social diseases."

Oral contraceptives, which have been widely available for less than 20 years, are the mainstay of many family planning programs (readers are referred to the relevant literature in obstetrics and endocrinology for details of the mechanisms of action of oral contraceptives). Oral contraceptives (OC's), which are generally used in the combined form (estrogen plus progestin), have very low failure rates (0.5-1.5) when taken as prescribed. They are also coitus-independent, usually very cheap, and can be used by a woman on her own initiative. However, they must be used according to a rigorous schedule on a regular basis, and occasional failure to adhere to this schedule can readily lead to pregnancy (the use of a calendar or formal schedule for pill-taking among illiterate women in developing countries was expected to present formidable problems, but in actual practice such women have usually been able to use OC's successfully and without difficulty). Further, OC's are not without side-effects (menstrual irregularity, headache, blood pressure elevation), which may interfere with their acceptability. Considerable concern has also been expressed about the relation between oral contraceptive use and serious adverse effects, particularly thromboembolic episodes, and there is an extensive literature on this subject.* However, it should be noted that the risk of

---

*See Connell, E.B.: "The pill revisited." Family Planning Perspectives 7(2):62-71.

death from thromboembolic disease associated with OC's is
extremely small compared to maternal mortality rates. In
western countries, there are 1-3 thromboembolic deaths per
100,000 women-years of OC use. In developing countries, preliminary evidence suggests that this disease-specific death
rate is even lower, whereas maternal mortality rates are as
high as 300-500/100,000 live births.

Intra-uterine devices (IUD's) are available in many forms and
have failure rates of only 1-3 per 100 woman-years. They must
be inserted by a trained health worker and may cause unusual
bleeding or cramping, or, infrequently, perforation of the
uterus or pelvic inflammatory disease. Spontaneous expulsion
also occurs in a small percentage of cases. The particular
advantages of IUD use are that it requires only one decision
by a woman regarding her current contraceptive practice, that
it is coitus-independent and does not interfere with sexual
activity, and that its effects are reversible (in well over
90% of cases) if an intentional pregnancy is later desired.

Sterilization and abortion are methods which are increasingly
important but which have both aroused considerable controversy.
Both require the intervention of trained health workers and
the application of surgical techniques. On the other hand,
both are highly effective and, when properly performed, very
safe. The obvious differences between these methods are that
compared to abortion, sterilization is performed before the
occurrence of an undesired pregnancy and may involve either
(or both) sexual partners. Sterilization, both male and female,
is rapidly becoming a major approach advocated in officially
sponsored FPP's, particularly in Asia. Until recently, the
major procedure available for female sterilization was post-
partum tubal ligation. Recently this has changed with the
development of new techniques for "interval procedures" performed at a time not related to pregnancy. These precedures
include: laparoscopy, culdoscopy, and minilaparotomy (mini-lap).
This latter procedure, using only a 3 cm. suprapubic incision,
can be readily performed on an outpatient basis under local
anesthesia, with minimal post-operative care and few complications.

n the case of abortion, there is great variation in the types of legal constraints.* However, recent data from studies in several different countries indicate that where induced abortions are both legal and readily available, women seeking repeat abortions (recidivists) may account for as much as 20-50% of all induced (elective) abortions. Thus in some settings, readily available abortions appear definitely to be used as a regular form of birth control. For example, in one large municipal hospital serving a low income urban area in the Eastern U.S., repeat abortions rose from 3% to 34% of the total annual number of abortions performed, within a few years following the legalization of abortion. In this instance, a large percentage of all abortions, and also of abortion recidivists, were unmarried women under age 25.

Questions:

a) Define "total fertility rate":

b) State, in your own words, how you would measure the "success" of a given contraceptive method:

c) List the five major contraceptive methods used in organized FPP's around the world:

---

*See Tietze,C., Murstein,M.C.: Induced Abortion: 1975 Factbook. Reports on Population/Family Planning, The Population Council, December 1975, especially pp. 6-13.

<u>SUGGESTED RESPONSES:</u>

a) Total fertility rate (TFR) is the sum of age-specific
fertility rates (live births per 1000 women per year)
for all women by single years of age between the ages
of 15 and 44 (see Unit III/7, p. 13). TFR represents
the hypothetical number of live births that would occur
per 1000 women of reproductive age if they all progressed
through their reproductive lives with the age-specific
fertility rates of a given year. TFR is thus a cross-
sectional measure of current fertility patterns. A TFR
of 2.0-2.2 would indicate a "replacement level" of
fertility, whereby the average married couple (2 persons)
is likely to produce approximately two children, a reproductive rate which would lead eventually to "zero
population growth" in a given society.

b) The success of a given contraceptive method, as we have
defined it above, can be expressed as:

1 - (no. of pregnancies per 100 woman-years of use).
For example, if in a group of women who all use oral
contraceptives regularly for a full year there are 3
pregnancies per 100 users, then the success of the pill
during this time period is:

$$1 - (3/100) = 0.97 \text{ (or 97\%)}$$

However, it should also be noted that many (perhaps
most) women of reproductive age are sexually active some
100 times per year. Thus, if a TFR of 2.0 is desired for
women completing their average reproductive age-span of
30 years, then an effective contraceptive method will
need to be used during all sexual exposures where there
is a substantial risk of pregnancy. If we assume 100
exposures per women-year x 30 years, this is 3,000 sexual
exposures per woman. Allowing for two periods each of
pregnancy (9 months) and lactation (9 months), during
which there is no real risk of further pregnancy, this

III/8, p. 10

*means that an effective contraceptive method will have
to be used successfully for 27 years per woman x 100
sexual exposures per year, or for some 2,700 sexual
exposures.*

c) *abortions (induced, legal)
condoms
IUD's
oral contraceptives
sterilization*

NATIONAL FAMILY PLANNING PROGRAMS

On a global scale, existing national family programs
(i.e., governmentally sponsored or public-sector programs)
are characterized by wide variations according to their
goals, their target populations, the particular combination
of contraceptive methods used, the degree to which these
programs attempt to meet expressed demands or to create
new demands by use of public education or specific incentives,
and their particular approaches to the systematic delivery
of family planning services.

Family planning programs are not a uniform set of activities.
Their existence in various countries has been largely
fashioned by prevailing sociocultural forces, local economics,
the infrastructure of basic health services (particularly
in rural areas), stated governmental policies, the general
level of socioeconomic development, recent demographic
trends in the age of marriage, cultural factors affecting
the role and status of women, and factors influencing the
motivation of women to seek, avoid or reject such services.

As of 1973, some 63 of 117 developing countries (representing
over 90% of the total developing world population) had
made explicit commitments to official family planning policies
or had allowed family planning services to be developed. In
32 of these 63 countries, population programs were designed to
reduce the population growth rate, as indicated in Table 1 on
the next page.

TABLE 1

DEVELOPING COUNTRIES, BY FAMILY PLANNING POLICY AND POPULATION SIZE, AS OF 1973

Population (millions)	Policy to reduce growth rate	Support to family planning, nondemographic reasons
100 and above	China India Indonesia	Brazil
50–100	Bangladesh Pakistan Mexico	Nigeria
25–50	Philippines Thailand Turkey Egypt South Korea Iran	
15–25	Colombia Morocco Taiwan	South Africa Zaire North Vietnam South Vietnam Afghanistan Sudan Algeria
10–15	Sri Lanka Kenya Nepal West Malaysia	Tanzania Venezuela Uganda Iraq Chile
Under 10	Ghana Tunisia Dominican Republic Hong Kong Laos Singapore Jamaica Trinidad & Tobago Mauritius Botswana Fiji Barbados Gilbert & Ellice	Cuba Khmer Ecuador Rhodesia Guatemala Mali Bolivia Haiti El Salvador Honduras Dahomey Paraguay Nicaragua Costa Rica Panama Liberia The Gambia

Reprinted with the permission of the Population Council from "The record of family planning programs," by Ronald Freedman and Bernard Berelson, Studies in Family Planning, volume 7, number 1 (January 1976), p. 5.

It is particularly noteworthy that almost all of the larger developing countries are included in Table 1, and that official pronouncements of family planning policies in these countries have been quite recent, dating in most cases from 1965 or later. Family planning policies and programs are thus both a recent and pervasive phenomenon in developing countries.

In schematic form, a national family planning program can be outlined as follows:

Family Planning Program

FPP =
| (1) policy & resource commitment | to | (2) delivery system | of | (3) contraceptive methods | to |

| (4) new acceptors | who | (5) continue use | → | (6) fertility regulation |

A thorough understanding of FPP's will require attention to each of the six major elements in this schematic outline. The section that follows is designed to help you interpret the extensive FPP literature.

"Acceptors" are usually defined as those in the target population, married women of reproductive age (MWRA) or their husbands, who enroll in officially sponsored programs during a calendar year. Assessment of FPP's is often presented in terms of numbers

of new acceptors, either as the number of acceptors per
year per total number of MWRA, or as the number of acceptors
per year per residual target population (MWRA minus current
contraceptive users). Data for 1973 from eight different
countries are shown in Table 2.

TABLE 2

| 1973 acceptors as percentage of: | | | | |
Residual target (MWRA minus users)	All MWRA	Country	Program users as percentage of MWRA	All users as percentage of MWRA
15.7	8.9	Taiwan	21	55
14.9	6.9	Hong Kong	27	55
13.4	9.5	South Korea	24.5	30.5
9.5	7.1	Thailand	17.7	24.8
7.9	5.7	Colombia	14	31
3.7	3.0	Egypt	16.8	20.5
3.2	2.7	Mexico	1.0	13.1
1.6	1.5	Morocco	2.4	6.2

Reprinted with the permission of the Population Council from
"The record of family planning programs," by Ronald Freedman
and Bernard Berelson, Studies in Family Planning, volume 7,
number 1 (January 1976), p. 6.

In addition to identifying new acceptors of family planning
services, it is also critical to consider how long new
acceptors actually continue to use the particular method
accepted.   Estimation of program performance by use of
acceptance rates must therefore be continually modified by
an estimation of continuation rates, usually done at yearly
intervals. In general, continuation rates for recent
acceptors of the pill and IUD are of the order of 60-70%
after one year and 50-60% after two years. On the other
hand, continuation rates for sterilization (both male and
female) are usually well over 95% after two years, since
in most cases sterilization is successful and not reversible.

It is important to remember that among all MWRA in any
country, many women may already be practicing contraception,

ither by traditional methods or by modern methods which
re readily available by other means (i.e. by use of pills,
UD's or condoms obtained from private physicians or
harmacists). Those responsible for assessing the impact
f national family planning programs may therefore need
consider both the "substitution effect" (extent of
fficial enrollment and inclusion as "acceptors" of MWRA
ho would have continued to use privately available
ontraceptive techniques on their own), and also the
indirect effect" (extent of new use of privately available
ontraceptive methods by MWRA who have learned about con-
raception but have not enrolled in official programs).
hese terms ("substitution effect" and "indirect effect")
re often used in reports on the effectiveness of family
lanning programs in a manner analogous to the use of
false positive" and "false negative" in the clinical
iterature, since these effects may distort the interpre-
ation of FPP-related contraceptive use rates as compared
o overall contraceptive use rates.

Referring back to Table 2, it is important to note the
ide variations between different countries in new acceptor
ates, FPP-related contraceptive use rates, and overall
ontraceptive use rates among MWRA. In Taiwan and Hong
ong, for example, the 1973 prevalence of total contracep-
ive use (or the "contraceptive use rate") was over 50%.
n both countries, data from field surveys showed that use
f contraception was widespread, whether or not contracep-
ive methods were obtained through the national FPP. In
oth countries, 1973 new acceptor rates were also high.
y contrast, in Mexico and Morocco, where new acceptance
ates were low, overall contraceptive use rates were also
ow. Possible inferences from these data are (1) that in
ountries where effective contraceptive methods were
lready available (from whatever sources), and where the
practice of contraception was generally viewed as socially
and culturally acceptable, national FPP's had a better
chance of success in reaching MWRA who were not yet

practicing contraception and family planning, whereas (2) in countries where the prior prevalence of contraceptive use was very low, there may have been greater sociocultural resistance to the introduction of contraceptive methods through official FPP's.

From the hypothetical data below, which country do you think illustrates the (a) substitution effect, (b) indirect effect on total contraceptive use rates?

COUNTRY X illustrates the _____ effect.

Year	New Acceptors (Percent of Residual MWRA)	All Users (Percent of all MWRA)
1973	9	16
1974	15	18
1975	21	25

- - - - - - - - - - - - - - - - - -

COUNTRY Y illustrates the _____ effect.

Year	New Acceptors	All Users
1973	2	6
1974	6	13
1975	9	25

COUNTRY X illustrates the substitution effect.
COUNTRY Y illustrates the indirect effect.

AN ILLUSTRATION

COUNTRY C has a total population of 50 million with a CBR of
40/1000, a TFR of 4.6/1000, and an annual PGR of 2.9%. An
Office of Family Planning has recently been established by
the Ministry of Health. Available data indicate that 10%
of all MWRA are currently practicing contraception. A health
worker is asked to plan an aggressive FPP that will enroll at
least 20% of the target population per year. How many women
would need to be enrolled in the FPP in the first year?

ANS: 1.3 million women, calculated as follows:
Population 50 million. Assume 50% female = 25 million.
Assume 55% of all females are age 15 or more = 13.75 million.
Assume 70% of adult females are between the ages of 15 - 44
= 0.70 x 13.75 = 9.5 million. If 10% are now practicing
contraception, some 8.5 million are "at risk." If 80% of
these 8.5 million adult women are married, then 0.8 x 8.5
million = 6.4 million married women now at risk. An enrollment of 20% of at-risk MWRA in the first year means enrolling
0.2 x 6.4 million = 1.28 million women. You will therefore
need to enroll some 1.3 million women in the first year of
your FPP in order to satisfy the expectations of your superiors.

These calculations are merely an exercise, and the various
assumptions in the above paragraph should be examined critically. However, you will probably be interested to know
that among the most successful FPP's, a new acceptor rate
of 15% per year (of the residual target population of MWRA)
is considered an excellent accomplishment. Even under these
circumstances, a continuing annual new acceptor rate of 15%
of previous non-users may only succeed in lowering the crude
birth rate (CBR) from 40/1000 to 30/1000 over a ten-year period.

The "30/30" guideline should be mentioned here. Some
demographers and family planning experts feel that in developing countries, a lowering of the crude birth rate below
30/1000 is closely tied to the achievement of at least a
30% level of regular contraceptive practice among all MWRA,
by whatever means. Given the fact that CBR in most countries
of Asia, Africa and Latin America is still closer to 40 than
to 30, the following table, based on a set of mathematical
models, is an illustrative example of the potential impact
of FPP's:

TABLE 3

Percentage new acceptors of nonusers annually	Fertility effect
15	About 10 points off CBR of 40–42 in 8 years, and stabilization there, with about 30% current use
10	About 6–7 points off, and stabilization, with about 25% current use
5	About 4 points off, and stabilization, with about 15% current use
2	Too small to measure

List at least three measures of performance which could be used to assess a given family planning program.

1._____

2._____

3._____

Performance measures for various aspects of a family planning program might include:

1.   *New acceptor rate as percent of all MWRA*
2.   *New acceptor rate as percent of residual target population*
3.   *Continuation rates (one year, two years, after two years), particularly for pill, IUD, condom*
4.   *Family planning program users as percent of all MWRA*
5.   *All contraceptive users as percent of all MWRA*
6.   *Success rate (1 - failure rate) for each contraceptive method employed*
7.   *Birth rate (crude and age-specific)*
8.   *Fertility rate (total and age-specific)*
9.   *Changes in population growth rate*
10. *Changes in patterns of child-spacing.*

APPROACHES TO FAMILY PLANNING

Up to this point we have concentrated mainly on particular contraceptive methods and on possible measures for evaluating FPP performance. We will now briefly consider some of the alternatives which exist in large-scale organization and delivery of family planning services. Many of these options can be encompassed by two questions: (1) Who does what? and (2) When and where do they do it?

WHO DOES WHAT?

In many developing countries, FPP's are now placing great emphasis on the roles of non-physicians in providing family planning services. For example, the Ministry of Public Health in Thailand in 1969 began a pilot program which permitted auxiliary midwives to prescribe oral contraceptives to women seeking family planning services. A simple

contraindication checklist" was used (Table 4) to identify
hose women who required direct referral to a physician for
pecial consultation and examination. Women who "passed"

TABLE 4

CHECKLIST FOR AUXILIARIES PROVIDING ORAL CONTRACEPTION

	Yes	No
History: ask if the patient has had a history of any of the following:		
Yellow skin or yellow eyes		
Mass in the breast		
Discharge from the nipple		
Swelling or severe pains in the legs		
Severe chest pains		
Unusual shortness of breath after exertion		
Severe headaches		
Excessive menstrual periods		
Increased frequency of menstrual periods		
Bleeding after sexual intercourse		
Examination: check the following:		
Yellow skin and yellow eye color		
Mass in the breast		
Nipple discharge		
Varicose veins in the legs		
Blood pressure (yes = above 160)		
Pulse (yes = above 120)		
Urine for sugar		
Urine for protein		

*Instructions: If all the above are answered in the negative, the patient may receive oral contraceptives, but, if any are answered in the positive, the patient must first be seen by a physician.

the checklist could be placed directly on oral contraceptives,
even without a pelvic examination. The decision to use
auxiliary midwives was based primarily on general recognition
of a severe shortage of physicians, particularly in rural
areas. Acceptance rates and continuation rates for oral

contraceptives were dramatically higher in the pilot program
in comparison to other areas of Thailand where paramedics
were not yet permitted to initiate contraceptive services.*
This pilot program has subsequently been expanded to include
large areas of rural Thailand. Similar efforts have also
been undertaken with apparent success in several countries
to demonstrate the feasibility and acceptance of IUD insertion by auxiliary personnel, without direct physician
supervision. It is possible that soon all forms of contraception which represent "medical intervention" (i.e. pills,
injectable contraceptives, IUD's, sterilizations and
abortions) will routinely be provided by medical auxiliaries
in the great majority of cases. Even in the United States,
there has been increasing reliance on nurse-midwives and
family planning nurse practitioners to provide education,
contraceptives and follow-up.

WHEN AND WHERE?

The immediate post-partum period has become recognized
within the last 15 years as a particularly good time for
active intervention directed toward general health education,
maternal and infant nutrition, and family planning. The
"post-partum approach" to family planning generally refers
to the routine availability of female sterilization or IUD
insertion while women are still in the hospital following
delivery or abortion, or within three months after discharge.
(Use of the pill for immediate post-partum use has usually
been avoided, due to possible interference with lactation.)
Aggressive campaigns to reach women during this period have
assumed major programmatic importance in countries where
large numbers of births occur in hospitals, usually in
urban areas. In many societies childbirth usually takes
place in the home, and large-scale family planning efforts

---

*See Rosenfield, A.G. and Limcharoen, C. Auxiliary midwife
prescription of oral contraceptives. Amer J Obstet Gynecol
14:942-949, 1972.

in the immediate post-partum period may not yet be feasible. However, demonstration projects have shown that integration of family planning services within the context of maternal and child health (MCH) services may be an effective approach in rural areas. In Thailand, for example, where domestic childbirth has been traditional in rural areas, newly constructed MCH centers in outlying provinces have immediately attracted women in large numbers for obstetrical care.* More important, acceptance rates for post-partum sterilization and IUD insertion have been remarkably high, approaching 50% of all deliveries in some cases.

More recently, emphasis has been placed on delivery of services at the village level in rural areas. Distribution of OC's and condoms is sometimes carried out by selected villagers, in some cases involving the distribution of contraceptives directly to each household. Experience with these community-based distribution programs is drawing increasing attention in Thailand and many other countries.

In summary, recent family planning efforts in Thailand are characterized by the following:

- Increasing use of auxiliary health personnel
- Reliance on multiple contraceptive methods
- Integration of family planning and MCH services
- Primary orientation to rural areas
- Village level distribution of family planning services (OC's and condoms)
- Vigorous post-partum intervention.

---

*Rosenfield, A.G., and Varakamin, S. The post-partum approach to family planning, Amer J Obstet Gynecol, 112:1-13, 1972.

OTHER COUNTRIES

Other countries illustrate additional features of large-
scale FPP's. In Colombia, an explicit government policy
is aimed at reducing fertility and also at giving every
married couple the right to decide the number and spacing of
their children.* There are three sizable FPP's, one operated
by the Ministry of Health, one by the Colombian Association
for Family Welfare (PROFAMILIA, a private organization affi-
liated with the International Planned Parenthood Federation),
and one by the Colombian Association of Medical Schools
(ASCOFAME), based primarily in university teaching hospitals.
Colombia, with an estimated total current population of 25
million, a CBR of 32/1000 and a crude death rate of some
10/1000, has an annual PGR of 22/1000, or 2.2%. Recent rural-to-urban migration has been dramatic, with nearly 50% of
the total population now living in towns of 20,000 or more
persons. ASCOFAME and PROFAMILIA have been active only for
some 12-15 years, and it was not until 1970 that an official
government policy on family planning was pronounced. (The influence of the Roman Catholic Church and the existence of a
traditional and conservative governmental bureaucracy must
be borne in mind.)

Recent government-sponsored activities in family planning
have involved arrangements with UNFPA (the United Nations
Fund for Population Activities) and also with PAHO (the
Pan American Health Organization). Government family planning
services are now an integral component of MCH services throughout the country. Government family planning services are
essentially free, utilizing oral contraceptives and IUD's in
that order, as the major methods of contraception (PROFAMILIA
and ASCOFAME rely much more heavily on the IUD). Some 40%
of Colombian women are now practicing contraception.

---

*See Sanin, E.P. Colombia. Country Profiles. The
Population Council, 1976.

In summary, the recent Colombian experience in family planning illustrates the following points:

- Concurrent involvement of the public and private sectors
- Extensive involvement of university medical centers
- Development of an official FPP in a conservative and traditional society
- Direct participation of international agencies.

India, with the world's second largest population (over 600 million), contains over 20% of the total population of all developing countries. India is unique in terms of its physical, geographic, ethnic, linguistic, and social diversity, and there is no way in one short paragraph to summarize adequately the development of its family planning services. India was the first non-Communist country to adopt an officially sponsored population policy (in 1951), and as of 1975 it led the world in the use of sterilization as a contraceptive method. In 1975 some 16% of all married Indian couples were regular contraceptive users. However, continuation of the current estimated PGR of 2.0% will lead to a population of some one billion persons by the year 2,000, and the Indian government has recently demonstrated an even more aggressive approach to birth control. Special attention has been given to the following efforts: condom distribution, a hospital-based post-partum intervention program, and a highly successful focus on male sterilization, by use of methods such as "vasectomy camps," often with specific financial incentives to those enrolling in the FPP. For any serious student of family planning services, India dramatizes, at each of the six steps in our schematic outline of a family planning program, the enormous complexity of achieving an effective national FPP in a large and heterogenous developing country.*

---

*See P. Visaria and A.R. Jain. India. Country Profiles. The Population Council, 1976.

Questions

1. Using the material presented in this unit and in III/7 (and any other information you may already have on the subject), list at least three factors that are likely to promote, and three factors that are likely to inhibit, the establishment of an effective national family planning program in a developing country.

FACTORS INHIBITING

(FI-a). _____

(FI-b). _____

(FI-c). _____

FACTORS PROMOTING

(FP-a). _____

(FP-b). _____

(FP-c). _____

2. Now, on the schematic FPP diagram below indicate the point at which each of these factors has its main effect. (You may wish to abbreviate your answers by using the corresponding letter designations).

III/8, p. 26

Factors Inhibiting (↓)

| (1) Policy and Resource Commitment | (2) Delivery System | (3) Contraceptive Methods | (4) New Acceptors | (5) Continue Use | (6) Fertility Regulation |

FPP = Commitment to System of Methods to Acceptors who

Factors Promoting (↑)

SUGGESTED RESPONSES

1. _You could have chosen any three of the following selections from each list:_

FACTORS INHIBITING FPP'S

(FI-a).   _Pro-natalist policies and attitudes_
(FI-b).   _Religious or legal opposition_
(FI-c).   _Insufficient budget and personnel_
(FI-d).   _Poor health care infrastructure_
(FI-e).   _Under-use of auxiliaries_
(FI-f).   _Childbirth usually at home_
(FI-g).   _No choice between contraceptives_
(FI-h).   _Target population unaware of FPP services_
(FI-i).   _Local customs and superstitions_
(FI-j).   _Side effects of contraceptive use_

FACTORS PROMOTING FPP'S

(FP-a).   _Explicit government policy supporting birth control_
(FP-b).   _Adequate budget for FPP_
(FP-c).   _Support from international agencies_
(FP-d).   _Solid health care infrastructure (especially in rural areas)_
(FP-e).   _Use of auxiliary health workers_
(FP-f).   _Post-partum intervention_
(FP-g).   _Ready availability of contraceptive methods_
(FP-h).   _Choice between contraceptives_
(FP-i).   _Educational/promotional campaigns_
(FP-j).   _Financial incentives_
(FP-k).   _Public awareness of contraceptive effectiveness._

2. FACTORS AFFECTING A FAMILY PLANNING PROGRAM

Factors Inhibiting (↓)

(FI-a) (FI-d) (FI-g) (FI-h) (FI-i)
(FI-b) (FI-e) (FI-i)
(FI-c) (FI-f)

FPP = Commitment to | System of | Methods to | Acceptors who

| (1) Policy and Resource | (2) Delivery System | (3) Contraceptive Methods | (4) New Acceptors | (5) Continue Use | (6) Fertility Regulation |

(FP-a) (FP-c) (FP-g) (FP-i) (FP-k)
(FP-b) (FP-d) (FP-h) (FP-j)
(FP-e)
(FP-f)

Factors Promoting (↑)

CONCLUSION

Many important aspects of Family Planning Services were not presented in this unit. Among others, they include the following:

- The relation between population growth and socioeconomic development
- The recent family planning activities in China
- The relation between formal education and use of family planning services
- Current pro-natalist attitudes in certain developing countries
- Current contraceptive research, including immunological approaches
- Family planning for unmarried persons
- Details of private sector activities in family planning
- The appropriate training and roles of physicians in FPP's.

There is an extensive literature on these issues and other aspects of family planning. In addition to the footnotes included within this unit, a list of suggested further reading is provided for your use.

SUGGESTED FURTHER READING

1. Berelson, B. World Population: Status Report 1974. Reports on Population/Family Planning. The Population Council 1974.

2. Dryfoos, J.G. The United States National Family Planning Program, 1968-74. Studies in Family Planning 7(3):80-92, 1976.

3. Freedman, R. and Berelson, B. The Record of Family Planning Programs. Studies in Family Planning 7(1):1-40, 1976.

4. Hemachudha, C. and Rosenfield, A.G. National Health Services and Family Planning: Thailand, a Case Study. Amer J Public Health 65:864-871, 1975.

5. Mauldin, W.P. Assessment of National Family Planning Programs in Developing Countries. Studies in Family Planning 6(2):30-36, 1975.

6. Omran, F.K. Family Planning Methods: Contraception, Abortion, and Sterilization. In Omran, A.O. (editor), Community Medicine in Developing Countries, Springer Publishing Co., 1974.

7. Robbins, J. Unmet Needs for Family Planning: A World Survey. Family Planning Perspectives 5(4):232-236, 1973.

8. Romm, F.J. et al. A Comparison of Program and Contraceptive Use Continuation Rates in a Family Planning Clinic. Amer J Public Health 65:693-699, 1975.

9. Rosenfield, A.G. Family Planning: An International Perspective. Ob/Gyn Digest, July 1974, pp. 13-20.

10.   Rosenfield, A.G., and Castadot, R.G.   Early Postpartum and Immediate Postabortion Intrauterine Contraceptive Device Insertion.   Amer J Obstet Gynecol 118:1104-1114, 1974.

11.   Rosenfield, A.G.   Family Planning Programs: Can More Be Done?   Studies in Family Planning 5(4):115-122, 1974.

12.   Watson, W.B., and Lapham, R.J. (editors).   Family Planning Programs: World Review 1974.   Studies in Family Planning 6(8):205-322, 1975.

13.   Wriggins, W.H., and Guyot, J.F. (editors).   Population, Politics and the Future of Southern Asia, Columbia University Press, 1973.

III/9: PROTEIN-CALORIE MALNUTRITION

BY

MICHAEL M. STEWART, M.D., M.P.H
ROBERT M. SUSKIND, M.D.

Contents

Note: The table below is included as general background information, although you will not necessarily need to refer to it while completing this Unit.

SUMMARY OF RECOMMENDED DAILY INTAKES

	Infant 0–11 months	Toddler 1–3 years (13 kg)	Preschool 4–6 years (18 kg)	School-Age Children			Adult Male	Adult Female		
				7–9 years (27 kg)	10–12 years (36 kg)	13–15 years (49 kg)	Male (63 kg)	Not Pregnant or Lactating (55 kg)	Pregnant third trimester	Lactating
Calories	110 (per kg body weight)	1,300	1,700	2,100	2,500	M 3,100 F 2,600	3,600	2,300	2,760	3,100
Protein (gms)	2.3–1.2 (per kg body weight)	14.3	17.5	24.9	31.0	41.1	46	39	45	54
Vitamin A: retinol (mcg)	300	250	300	400	575	725	750	750	750	750
B-Carotene (mcg)	600	500	600	800	1,150	1,450	1,500	1,500	1,500	1,500
Vitamin D (mcg)	10	10	10	2.5	2.5	2.5	2.5	2.5	10	10
Vitamin B$_{1}$ (mcg)	0.3	0.9	1.5	1.5	2.0	2.0	2.0	2.0	3.0	2.5
Thiamine (mg)	0.4	0.5	0.7	0.8	1.0	M 1.2 F 1.0	1.3	0.9	1.1	1.2
Riboflavin (mg)	0.6	0.7	0.9	1.2	1.4	M 1.7 F 1.4	1.8	1.3	1.6	1.8
Niacin equivalents (mg)	6.6	8.6	11.2	13.9	16.5	M 20.4 F 17.2	21.1	15.2	18.2	20.4
Ascorbic Acid (mg)	20	20	20	20	20	30	30	30	50	50
Iron (mg)	10	10	10	10	10	24	10	28	28	28
Calcium (mg)	500–600	400–500	400–500	400–500	600–700	600–700	400–500	400–500	1,000–1,200	1,000–1,200

Source: Adapted from *Health Aspects of Food and Nutrition* (FAO/WHO, 1969).

INTRODUCTION

Hundreds of millions of persons throughout the world are malnourished, perhaps as many as 25% of the world population. The population groups at greatest risk, particularly in deprived socioeconomic areas, are infants and young children, and pregnant and lactating women. Persons with certain chronic diseases are also especially vulnerable. In developed countries, various types of "malnutrition of affluence" have become special problems. In a more limited way, food faddism has led to specific nutrient deficiencies in certain groups.

On a global scale, some 100 million children under 5 years of age are seriously affected by malnutrition. In Latin American cities, a recent study revealed that malnutrition was associated, directly or indirectly, with more than 50% of all deaths in children under 5. Various prevalence surveys conducted during the past 10-15 years in different countries of Asia, Africa and Latin America have identified between 20% and 35% of children as being moderately to severely malnourished, as shown in Table 1.

Table 1

Range and Median of Percent Prevalence of PCM in Community Surveys[a]

Area	Number of communities	Number of surveys	Number of children examined	Severe forms Range	Severe forms Median	Moderate forms Range	Moderate forms Median
Latin America	8	11	108,715	0.5–6.3	1.6	3.5–32.0	18.9
Africa	5	7	24,739	1.7–9.8	4.4	5.4–44.9	26.5
Asia	4	7	39,494	1.1–20.0	3.2	16.0–46.4	31.2
Total	17	25	172,948	0.5–20.0	2.6	3.5–46.4	18.9

[a] *Selected surveys with more than 1000 children examined.*

Source: J. M. Bengoa in Protein-Calorie Malnutrition. Academic Press, 1975. Reprinted with permission.

Primary protein-calorie malnutrition (PCM) is the most frequent and devastating nutritional problem in areas where
the overall nutritional environment is poor; that is, where
the availability of essential foods is limited, where the
typical diet contains inadequate amounts and ratios of
basic nutrients and where crowding and inadequate sanitation
lead to an increased frequency of infectious diseases. An
example of a poor nutritional environment is given in the
following vignette on village life on rural Guatemala:

"The typical Mayan Indian home of the highlands illustrates
the contribution physical environment makes to causality
of malnutrition. Cooking was over an open fire on the
floor; only 10% of village families had a stove. There was
no water faucet and no pump; water was carried on the head
in earthen jars from a communal source.

In a region where everything grows -- even the fence posts
sprout leaves in the rainy season -- the choice of basic
foods was culturally restricted to corn and beans, morning,
noon, and night. Fruits and vegetables were cash crops.
An animal census of the villages showed few sources of
animal protein and especially of milk for toddlers and young
children. Cows existed but were scarce. As features of the
social environment, tradition, custom, and taboos strongly
influenced the choice of foods in a land of potential
plenty. The biological environment also contributed to a
faulty nutritional state through poor sanitation in the
storage and preparation of food." (Gordon, J. E., ref. 12)

PCM, which frequently occurs in settings such as the one
described, has multiple adverse consequences, both for
individuals and society as a whole. These include (among
others) increased childhood morbidity and mortality, diminished resistance to infection, and impairment of psychomotor
development.

The nutritional fate of millions of persons is, of course, closely tied to major socioeconomic issues such as stages of national economic development, import-export ratios, patterns of population growth, increasing human use of animal rather than plant foods, uncertainties regarding the current status and future prospects of the fishing and agricultural industries, and patterns of international cooperation in food-related trade as well as in stockpiling and sharing of food reserves. These large-scale world food issues are beyond the scope of this unit, but they should be pursued by any student seriously interested in nutrition, food production and food distribution on an international scale.*

Although primary PCM is now rarely seen in clinics or on hospital wards in the United States, secondary forms, both in children and adults, occur far more frequently than is generally appreciated, due to various renal, gastrointestinal, neurologic, cardiopulmonary, neoplastic and other diseases. There are three major mechanisms which contribute to the occurrence of both primary and secondary malnutrition: deficient nutrient intake, increased nutrient requirements, and increased nutrient losses. Various combinations of these mechanisms (as well as others) are found in all patients with either primary or secondary PCM.

Many hospitalized patients have unrecognized (and therefore untreated) nutritional problems. Moreover, it is widely felt that clinical nutrition receives too little emphasis in the medical school curriculum. The nutritional assessment of patients is not sufficiently stressed and may be superficial or incomplete. Moreover, the nutritional aspects of chronic diseases and the relationship between a patient's living environment and nutritional status is often overlooked by the physician. The general problem of malnutrition therefore has direct clinical relevance in the education of medical students and other health professionals in all geographic areas.

---

*See, for example, Nutrition and Agricultural Development, N.S. Scrimshaw and M. Behar, Editors, Plenum Press, 1976. Also, reference 2 deals with the special problem of famine.

This unit addresses selected issues related to the occurrence and ecological determinants of malnutrition, particularly PCM in its primary and secondary forms. The general goals are:

1. To describe various methods used to assess the nutritional status of individuals and population groups.

2. To emphasize the magnitude of the worldwide problem of primary childhood PCM, as well as its major clinical, biochemical, and immunologic features.

3. To review the nutritional implications of other primary disease states.

4. To identify elements in the biological, physical and social environment which contribute to the occurrence of PCM.

5. To indicate opportunities for prevention and early detection of PCM.

OBJECTIVES

At the completion of this unit, you will be able to:

1. List at least three techniques used to assess nutritional status.

2. Summarize the major differences between two severe forms of PCM, marasmus and kwashiorkor.

3. Explain the major interactions between malnutrition, infection, and the immune response.

4. List at least three possible ways to reduce the frequency and severity of PCM.

PROTEIN-CALORIE MALNUTRITION: ASSESSMENT AND CLASSIFICATION

In a broad conceptual sense, there are four major types of malnutrition:

1) Primary protein-calorie malnutrition.

2) Secondary malnutrition (e.g. malnutrition associated with another primary disease state).

3) Specific mineral and vitamin deficiencies (e.g. iron, iodine and Vitamin A deficiency).

4) Overnutrition (e.g. obesity, hyperlipidemia, and hypervitaminosis).

We are particularly concerned here with **primary and** secondary malnutrition.* In developing countries, patterns of infant and second-year mortality are closely associated with the frequency of PCM. PCM and infection, interacting synergistically, together represent the single greatest threat to health for the world's children.

Primary PCM in infancy and childhood is usually classified quantitatively on two scales, one of severity (mild-moderate-severe) and one of chronicity (acute vs. chronic). The severity of PCM is assessed primarily in terms of deficits in expected weight-for-age, using as a reference standard the weight of the 50th percentile of children in a healthy control population in Europe or North America, or in some cases, a well-nourished local population group. (The most widely used reference point is the so-called "Harvard standard.") Contrary to popular assumptions, there is little evidence for major genetic differences in growth potential during the first year or two of life among most groups of

*Students particularly interested in problems of mineral and vitamin deficiency may wish to consult references 10, 19 & 20.

of children in different ethnic, geographic and social settings. Although this may seem surprising, numerous studies have shown that it is usual for well-nourished infants and children in developing countries to follow closely the same growth curves as infants and children in developed countries. As a result, the severity of PCM can be classified into three groups defined by the patient's weight expressed as a percentage of the 50th percentile of the Harvard standard:

Degree of PCM	% Expected Weight-for-Age
first-degree	75% - 90%
second-degree	60% - 75%
third-degree	under 60%

A typical weigh-for age growth use in Colombia is shown in Figure 1 on the next page.* Such growth charts serve two major purposes: 1) classification of groups of children according to nutritional status, and 2) early identification of individual children whose growth is substandard and who are, by definition, malnourished.

The use of weight-for-age as a measure of nutritional status, however, does not permit ready differentiation between acute malnutrition and chronic malnutrition. These are more clearly distinguished by measurements of weight-for-height (for acute PCM) and height-for-age (for chronic PCM). Specifically, weight-for-age measurements do not take into account the concomitant height deficit (or stunting) which accompanies prolonged childhood malnutrition (see reference 18). Therefore, as a measurement of linear growth, height-for-age (which is the patient's height expressed as a percentage of the 50th percentile of the Harvard standard) is used to classify grades of chronic malnutrition:

---

*Note that in Figure 1, first-degree PCM is defined as 75-85% of expected weight for age, rather than 75-90%.

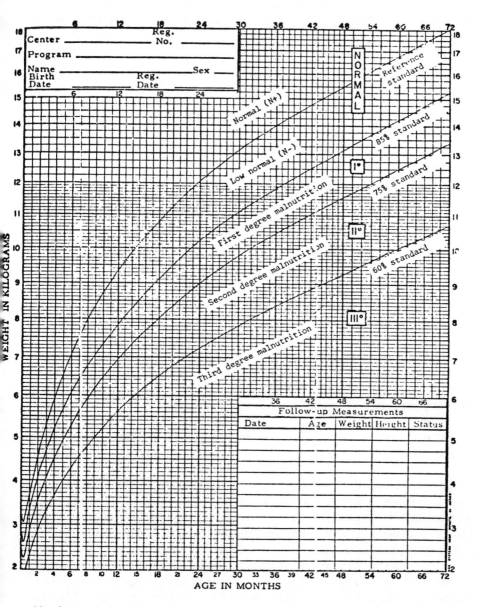

Fig. 1. Graph for Classification of Nutritional Status in Children Under Six

Source: Joe D. Wray and Alfredo Aguirre, "Protein Calorie Malnutrition in Candelaria, Colombia—I. Prevalence; Social and Demographic Causal Factors," *Journal of Tropical Pediatrics*, Vol. 15 (1969), pp. 76–98.

Degree of Chronic PCM	% Expected Height-for-Age
Grade I	90 - 95%
Grade II	85 - 90%
Grade III	under 85%

Measurement of the deficit of weight-for height (which is the patient's weight as a percentage of the 50th percentile of weight for children of the same height) is used to assess the degree of acuteness of PCM (often referred to as wasting):

Degree of Acute PCM	% Expected Weight-for-Height
Grade I	80 - 90%
Grade II	70 - 80%
Grade III	under 70%

These three measures - weight-for-age, height-for-age, and weight-for-height - are important tools for detecting PCM in individual children, for monitoring their growth over time, and for classifying groups of children with PCM by degree of severity and chronicity. The above measures can be augmented by additional techniques such as mid-arm circumference and triceps skinfold thickness.

Such techniques of nutritional anthropometry, which include measurements of weight, height, arm circumference, skinfold thickness, and a number of others, are widely used in conducting community nutrition surveys, since they are relatively simple and cheap, and require only modest technical expertise and a minimum of specialized equipment (scale, tape-measure, skinfold calipers). The use of nutritional anthropometry in field surveys, as well as in clinical settings, can help to identify early growth deficits, often well before PCM has become clinically evident. In addition, the measurement of weight-for-height also permits identification and classification of PCM even when a child's age is not obtainable.

This can be particularly helpful in places where birth-
dates are not recorded and where children's precise
chronological ages are unknown, a situation most likely
to occur in the rural areas of many developing countries
where the risk of PCM is especially high.

In addition to anthropometry, certain biochemical and
hematological indices are used in nutritional assessment.
These include: total serum proteins, albumin, transferrin
(i.e., total iron-binding capacity), and retinol-binding
protein, all of which reflect the adequacy of visceral protein
synthesis; 24-hour urinary creatinine, to evaluate lean
body mass; hemoglobin and hematocrit; and a variety of
assays to determine vitamin and mineral status. X-rays are
also used to evaluate bone age and bony abnormalities, for
example, as seen in rickets caused by Vitamin D deficiency.
Physiological measurements may be used, such as testing for
dark-adaptation in order to detect "night-blindness", an
early manifestation of Vitamin A deficiency.

MARASMUS AND KWASHIORKOR

Important distinctions can be made between the two most
severe forms of PCM, marasmus and kwashiorkor, both of which
are considered to be third-degree malnutrition. Both forms
of severe PCM have been preceded by mild (first-degree) and
moderate (second-degree) states, which, if they had been
detected earlier, could have been prevented from progressing
to the more severe forms. This progression from mild to
severe is shown in Figure 2. Marasmus is preceded by a long
period of increasing deficits in both weight and height,
whereas kwashiorkor (see below) is preceded by gradual
reduction in serum proteins. Marasmus results from prolonged
dietary deficiencies of calories, protein, vitamins and minerals. Severe wasting and stunting may both be present.

FIG. 2   LINES OF DEVELOPMENT IN PROTEIN-CALORIE MALNUTRITION OF EARLY CHILDHOOD

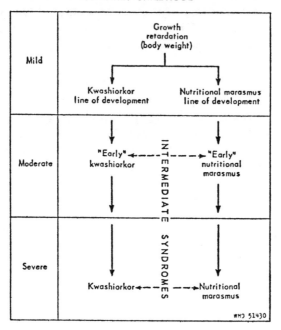

The diagram is a schematic attempt to correlate the development of mild, moderate and severe protein-calorie malnutrition in the two main lines of development—i.e., leading to kwashiorkor and to nutritional marasmus as well as to indeterminate, atypical, intermediate syndromes. The dotted lines stress the potential convertibility from one line of development to the other .

(see reference 6)

Examination of a marasmic child reveals emaciation, disappearance of body fat, and loss of lean body mass (i.e., muscle mass). There is often evidence of psychomotor retardation or apathy , and there may be clinical evidence of specific vitamin deficiencies, such as xerophthalmia (Vitamin A deficiency) or rickets (Vitamin D deficiency).

Marasmus usually occurs in the first year of life, following early cessation or inadequacy of breast-feeding and the introduction of nutritionally poor weaning or post-weaning foods such as dilute artificial milk or a thin gruel. The occurrence of marasmus may be hastened by frequent bouts of infection. Despite the obviously severe clinical findings, biochemical abnormalities in marasmus may be minimal. For example, levels of serum albumin, transferrin and retinol-binding protein may be relatively normal. Marasmus can be considered most simply as the consequence of severe and prolonged childhood starvation.

Kwashiorkor, on the other hand, is a severe form of PCM which usually occurs somewhat later in childhood, in the second or third year of life. It is assoicated with a readily detectable imbalance between dietary protein and carbohydrate intake, with a significantly reduced protein-to-to-carbohydrate ratio. In addition, the onset of kwashiorkor is usually precipitated by one or more episodes of infection, most often diarrheal and respiratory diseases (malaria, where endemic, may play a major role in PCM). There are several mechanisms by which infection interacts with nutritional states leading to kwashiorkor. These include: anorexia (which reduces food intake); changes in food offered to an infant or child during illness (such as withholding solid food); increased metabolic losses; decreased nutrient absorption (especially in gastrointestinal infections); internal sequestration or wastage of nutrients; and the effects of certain medications (for example, purgatives). The child with kwashiorkor presents clinically with edema, severe muscle wasting, hepatomegaly with fatty infiltration of the liver, and decreases in serum albumin, total iron-binding capacity and retinol-binding protein. In addition, psychomotor and affective changes are common, such as irritability, apathy, indifference to environmental stimuli, and withdrawal. Dermatoses and marked pigmentary changes of the hair are frequent. Biochemical abnormalities observed in children with kwashiorkor include: reduced levels of serum albumin and other serum proteins, reduction in total and essential amino acids, and reduction in other nutrients such as iron and Vitamin A. Kwashiorkor occurs when weaning foods (foods used to supplement breast milk, before the complete cessation of breast-feeding) contain adequate calories

but too little protein. This most often occurs in settings
where low-protein cereals (such as glutinous rice), starchy
roots (such as cassava), tubers (such as yams), or fruits
(such as plaintain) are used as the major food source in the
weaning and post-weaning diet. Inadequate protein intake,
plus recurrent and inadequately treated infections, leads
to kwashiorkor.

Many malnourished children present with intermediate or
combined forms of PCM which are classified as "marasmic
kwashiorkor." They are equally as sick as children with
"pure" forms of PCM, and the clinical and biochemical findings
include various combinations of the descriptions given above.

For the nutritional assessment of individual children over
relatively short time periods, it is critical to note the
trend and velocity of gains or losses in weight, in addition
to the absolute value of weight in terms of a reference
standard. Figure 3, for example, shows the weight curve of
a previously well-nourished child who developed kwashiorkor
at age 30 months, as compared to the weight curve of another
child gradually recovering from marasmus which had its onset
in the first year of life.

Figure 3

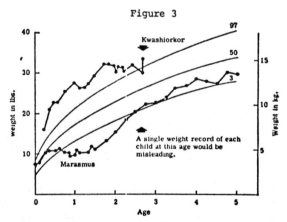

*Comparison of the weight curves of two children with kwashiorkor and marasmus.
The mother of the marasmic child was being congratulated for a good gain along
the third centile while the child on the ninety-seventh centile was being
admitted to hospital with kwashiorkor.*

Source: D. Morley. Paediatric Priorities in the Developing World.
Butterworths, 1973. Reprinted with permission.

In addition to growth retardation, PCM is closely associated with increased incidence and severity of infectious diseases, as noted above. The epidemiological interrelations of PCM and infectious diseases have been referred to as the "Malnutrition-Morbidity-Mortality Complex" (see Wray, ref.12). Poor nutrition increases susceptibility to common infections (such as diarrhea, upper and lower respiratory tract infections, measles, whooping-cough, chicken pox, etc.) and recurrent episodes of these infections further aggravate an already poor nutritional status and may precipitate acute PCM. Figure 4 illustrates the close relationship in one child's growth curve between repeated episodes of infectious disease and the adverse effect on childhood growth, manifested in this case by severe kwashiorkor. (Note that the reference standard for "normal" growth in Figure 4 is based on the healthy local childhood population.)

Figure 4

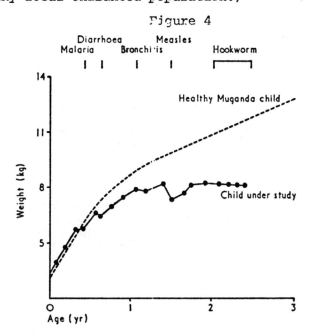

Effects of serial infections on the growth of a rural Ugandan child.

Source: A.G. Shaper et al (eds.), Medicine in a Tropical Environment. British Medical Association, 1972. Reprinted with permission.

Fortunately, evidence from a variety of field studies indicates that proper immunizations and prevention or reduction of the incidence of infectious diseases can also reduce the frequency of PCM. Moreover, direct efforts to improve nutritional status with proper supplementary feedings during and after weaning can also reduce the frequency and severity of episodes of common infectious diseases, as suggested in Table 2.

Table 2

Reduction in Diarrhea During Successive Three-Month Periods in Children in an Ambulatory Nutrition Supplementation/Education Program Colombia, 1964–1965

Age Groups (months)	Nutritional Status at Start of Program	Number of Episodes of Diarrhea Per Three-Month Period			
		First	Second	Third	Fourth
0–35	Mild PCM	1.49	1.04	0.77	0.64
	Moderate–Severe	1.86	0.82	0.97	0.63
36–72	Mild PCM	0.71	0.82	0.61	0.29
	Moderate–Severe	0.71	0.46	0.29	0.18

Source: Joe D. Wray, *Malnutrition and Diarrhea: The Evidence from Candelaria* (unpublished thesis; Chapel Hill, N.C.: University of North Carolina School of Public Health, 1967). Reprinted with permission of the author.

One of the most worrisome aspects of PCM is its possible impact on brain development and the eventual cognitive function and potential for effective social and economic contributions of affected children. The physical impact of PCM on intracranial space is shown in Figure 5. The precise relationship

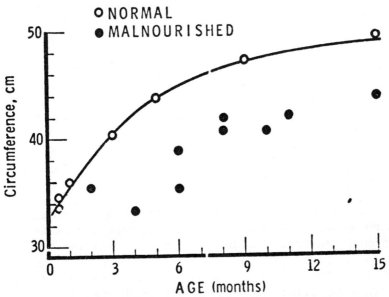

Figure 5

HEAD CIRCUMFERENCE VS POSTNATAL AGE

Winick, M. and Rosso, P. Head circumference and cellular growth of the brain in normal and marasmic children. J Pediat 74:774-778, 1969. Reprinted with permission.

between infant and childhood nutrition, brain development, and adult intellectual capacity and performance is an area of active current investigation, with suggestive but inconclusive results. However, since fetal and infant malnutrition are clearly associated with a decreased number and size of neurons, the long term effects of early PCM seem likely to include some degree of impaired mental and/or neurologic capacity among survivors.

MALNUTRITION AND THE IMMUNE SYSTEM

Recent studies have helped to elucidate the effect of malnutrition on various components of the human immune response
system (see reference 17 for details). In most children
with severe malnutrition, there is depression of cellular
immunity, as demonstrated by the decreased reactivity to skin
test antigens such as monilia, streptokinase-streptodornase,
and PPD. There are also decreased numbers of circulating
T-cells, and a decrease in lymphocyte reactivity to mitogens
and antigens in standard in vitro tests. Although total
immunoglobulins are usually normal or elevated in PCM, malnourished children often fail to develop normal antibody
responses to certain specific antigenic stimuli, such as
typhoid vaccine. The phagocytic function of polymorphonuclear
leucocytes (PMN's) is relatively intact. Some studies have
detected deficits in the ability of PMN's to kill ingested
bacteria, while other studies have found this phagocytic
killing function to be normal. In severely malnourished
children, the complement system is compromised, as measured
by reduced levels of circulating complement proteins, and
reduced hemolytic activity.

As a result of these several adverse effects of malnutrition
on the immune system, as well as the fact that the normal
immune response system in infants and young children may
not yet be fully developed, a child with PCM is particularly
susceptible to recurrent infections, which themselves then
lead to further deterioration of nutritional status.

SECONDARY PROTEIN-CALORIE MALNUTRITION

Children and adults with such primary diseases as cancer, chronic renal disease, chronic lung disease, cystic fibrosis and many other pathologic conditions may become severely malnourished and develop clinical findings and biochemical abnormalities which are characteristic of primary PCM. The patient with cancer exemplifies the problem of secondary malnutrition. Malnutrition may develop as a result of the neoplasm itself (a rapidly growing neoplasm consumes nutrients, for example) or because of the therapy being used. Prior to therapy, there may be anorexia, cancer cachexia, mechanical obstruction of the GI tract, malabsorption of ingested nutrients, or protein-losing enteropathy. The various types of therapy used -- surgery, chemotherapy, and radiation -- may also affect nutritional status. For example, surgery on a segment of the GI tract may interfere with nutrient ingestion and/or absorption. Chemotherapy and radiation can both cause anorexia, nausea, vomiting and diarrhea, as well as malabsorption. Various combinations of these different nutritional insults can affect the patient with cancer to such a degree that secondary malnutrition becomes a major clinical problem.

TREATMENT

Treatment of PCM is basically dietary. Protein, calories, vitamins and minerals must be provided in sufficient amounts to reverse the deficits in weight and/or height and also to allow for a substantial period of "catch-up growth". Caloric intake must be sufficient to allow good utilization of ingested protein. In most malnourished children a daily allowance of 150-160 cal./kg and 3-4 gm of protein/kg will be needed. Protein may be either of animal or vegetable origin. Many children with PCM require hospitalization when first seen, often because of intercurrent infection or sepsis, or because of serious fluid and electrolyte problems. These problems must be controlled before the long period of improved

III/9, p. 19

dietary treatment can be effectively begun.

One of the major challenges in the treatment of severe PCM is to find ways to return children "cured" of clinical PCM to their home environments with a significantly diminished probability of disease recurrence. Treatment in the hospital must therefore be accompanied by investigation of the ecological circumstances which allowed PCM to develop, and an effort to intervene , where possible to reduce the risk of recurrent PCM. This may include initiation or completion of childhood immunizations; education of the mother in proper breast-feeding or supplementary feeding practices; or provision of a protein-rich food supplement such as dried skim milk to be used in the home. The mortality rate among hospitalized children with severe PCM is high, primarily because of infection. For children who recover, the major challenge is to combine dietary treatment with preventive activities. Treatment for children with mild or moderate PCM consists primarily of food supplements and regular monitoring of growth and development. These services should be provided as close to the home as possible. It should be recognized that the mother is the key person in nutritional rehabilitation. If she fails to understand, accept or comply with the necessary treatment measures, reversal of PCM is unlikely.

PREVENTION

Strategies for prevention of PCM on a community-wide basis are simple in concept but may be extremely difficult to carry out. The two fundamental goals of preventive programs are 1) provision of a daily diet with adequate amounts and proportions of protein, calories, vitamins and minerals, and 2) reduction of the frequency and severity of infections. The methods used to achieve these goals may vary widely with the environmental, cultural and socioeconomic setting.

Breast milk is an excellent source of nutrition for most
children during the first 4-6 months of life, and the suckling
infant benefits in many additional ways from breast-feeding.
For example, breast milk provides several avenues of protection against infectious diseases; the breast is a source
of psychological security; and the availability of physically
close infant-maternal contact and early learning experiences
is ensured by suckling. It is important to note that in
most countries, weaning, or the separation of a child from
the mother's breast, is a process rather than an event.
The normal weaning process may last for 1-2 years, as shown
in Figure 6. However, supplementary foods will need to
be introduced while the child is still suckling, usually by
age six months.

Figure 6

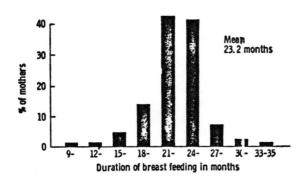

Study on duration of breast feeding in 291 mothers in a West African village.

Source: D. Morley. Paediatric Priorities in the Developing World.
Butterworths, 1973. Reprinted with permission.

There are many types of protein-rich food supplementation
programs. Some are based in local health centers, nutrition
centers or day care centers. Some distribute food supplements directly to the home. In many countries, feeding
programs for children and education programs for mothers
are components of an integrated program providing all basic

health services to the children in a community.* One of the
major challenges in many areas is to create a clear recognition within the community (particularly on the part of the
women) that malnutrition exists, that it is a problem, and
that it can be reversed or prevented. Many nutrition programs
focus on new mothers as a special target, since PCM in
children under five could theoretically be eliminated in a
community within five years if every young mother were
properly educated in breast-feeding, supplemental feeding, and
child care, and if infants and children were kept under
careful nutritional surveillance during the vulnerable
early years of life.**

Methods to reduce the frequency and severity of infections
involves many different types of activities.   It
must again be underscored that routine childhood immunizations will help greatly. Most important of all, however,
adequate nutrition during the weaning and post-weaning
period will reduce the number of episodes of common infections and thus prevent the continuation of the reciprocating
malnutrition-infection interaction.

---

*See Morley's discussion of "The Under-Fives' Clinic,"
 Chapter 19 in reference 9.

**See reference 21 for a detailed discussion of
  surveillance.

UNIT REVIEW

. List three types of measurement used to assess the
nutritional status of a child or a group of children
suspected of being malnourished.

a.

b.

c.

III/9, p. 23

2. State the major differences between marasmus and kwashiorkor in terms of:

a. Nutrient intake:

b. Nutritional anthropometry:

c. Biochemical measurements:

. Describe the major factors involved in the reciprocal interaction between malnutrition and infection in children:

1. *You should have included any three of the following measurements:*

   a. *nutritional anthropometry, especially including weight-for-age, height-for-age, weight-for-height, mid-arm circumference, triceps skinfold thickness.*

   b. *biochemical determinants, especially including the various serum proteins.*

   c. *hematological indices.*

   d. *clinical examination for signs of marasmus, kwashiorkor and vitamin or mineral deficiency.*

2. a. *nutrient intake:*

   (1) Marasmus results from prolonged dietary deficiencies of calories, proteins, vitamins and minerals.

   (2) Kwashiorkor results from protein-carbohydrate imbalance with reduced protein-carbohydrate ratio .

   b. *nutritional anthropometry:*

   (1) Marasmus - decreased weight-for-age , height-for-age, and normal weight-for-height.

   (2) Kwashiorkor - decreased weight-for-age and weight-for-height with relatively normal height-for-age.

   c. *biochemical measurements*

   (1) Marasmus - relatively normal serum proteins

   (2) Kwashiorkor - decreased serum proteins.

3. *Your response should have included most of the following factors:*

a. PCM occurs primarily at a period of life when the child's immune system is not yet fully developed.

b. PCM is associated with deficits in many components of the immune response: cellular immunity, specific antibody deficiencies, impaired bactericidal activity of phagocytes, and impaired complement activity.

c. PCM occurs in settings where crowding and poor hygiene increases the transmission of infectious agents.

d. Infection may decrease nutrient intake, increase nutrient requirements and increase nutrient losses.

REFERENCES

1. Berg, A. and Muscat, R. An Approach to Nutrition Planning. Amer. J. Clin. Nutrition 25:939-954, 1972 (analysis of large-scale governmental nutrition planning efforts).

2. Blix, G. et. al., Editors. Famine: Nutrition and Relief Operations in Times of Disaster. Uppsala, Sweden: Almquist and Wiksells, 1971 (Report of a 1970 Symposium of the Swedish Nutrition Foundation).

3. Christakis, G., Editor. Nutritional Assessment in Health Programs. Washington, D. C.: American Public Health Association, 1974 (concise paperback manual on assessment methods for different age groups).

4. Gordon, J. E. Social Implications of Nutrition and Disease. Arch. Environ. Health 18:216-234, 1969 (important reference article).

5. Harfouche, J. K. The Importance of Breast-feeding. J. Tropical Pediatrics. 16:133-175, 1970 (important reference article).

6. Jelliffe, D. B. The Assessment of the Nutritional Status of the Community. Geneva: WHO, 1966 (classic monograph, with considerable detail).

7. Jelliffe, D. B. Infant Nutrition in the Tropics and Subtropics. Geneva: WHO, 1968 (monograph oriented toward clinical practice).

8. Mata, L. J. Malnutrition-Infection Interactions in the Tropics. Amer. J. Trop. Med. Hyg. 24:564-574, 1975 (review article with much original data).

9. Morley, D. Paediatric Priorities in the Developing World. London: Buttersworths, 1973 (especially Chapters 6-13, dealing with infant feeding, growth, and various pediatric infections).

10. Nutrition Reviews: Present Knowledge in Nutrition (4th Edition). New York: The Nutrition Foundation, 1976 (summary of current clinical and biochemical information).

11. Olson, R. E., Editor. Protein-Calorie Malnutrition. New York: Academic Press, 1975 (biochemically-oriented report of a 1973 symposium held in Thailand).

12. Omran, A. R., Editors. Community Medicine in Developing Countries. New York: Springer, 1974 (useful overview chapters on nutrition and community health, MCH services and the malnutrition-morbidity-mortality complex).

13. Scrimshaw, N. W. Ecological Factors in Nutritional Disease. Amer. J. Clin. Nutrition 14:112-122, 1964 (important reference article).

14. Scrimshaw, N. S., Taylor, C. E., and Gordon, J. E. Interactions of Nutrition and Infection. Geneva: WHO, 1968 (classic reference work).

15. Shaper, A. G. et al, Editors. Medicine in a Tropical Environment. London: British Medical Association, 1972 (clinically oriented manual).

16. Stein, Z., et al. Famine and Human Development: The Dutch Hunger Winter of 1944-1945. New York: Oxford University Press, 1975 (epidemiological analysis of the effects of malnutrition on a cohort of children).

17 Suskind, R. M., Editor. Malnutrition and the Immune Response. New York: Raven Press, 1977 (recent reference in a rapidly expanding field).

18. Waterlow, J. C. Classification and Definition of Protein-Calorie Malnutrition. Brit. Med. Journal 3:566-569, 1972 (important reference article).

19. WHO: <u>Control of Nutritional Anemia with Special Reference to Iron Deficiency</u>, Technical Report Series No. 580. Geneva: WHO, 1975 (compact and valuable overview).

20. WHO: <u>Vitamin A Deficiency and Xerophthalmia</u>. Technical Report Series No. 590. Geneva: WHO, 1976 (compact and valuable overview).

21. WHO: <u>Methodology of Nutritional Surveillance</u>. Technical Report Series No. 593. Geneva: WHO, 1976 (important summary of environmental and social determinants of nutritional status and of various quantitative indices used in surveillance).

22. Winick M. <u>Malnutrition and Brain Development</u>. New York: Oxford University Press, 1976 (recent reference in a specialized field).